THE ANSWER MODEL:
A new path to healing

D1572270

John Montgomery, Ph.D. & Todd Ritchey

TAM Books

© 2010 TAM Books
A division of The Answer Model
Santa Monica, CA, USA
All Rights Reserved
Unauthorized Reproduction of this Document is Prohibited

Cover Design by Helen Shardray and John Montgomery

ISBN 978-0-9822960-1-1

photograph of lemur by Quentin
Bloxam; graciously provided by Noel
Rowe, from *The Pictorial Guide to the
Living Primates*, Pogonias Press

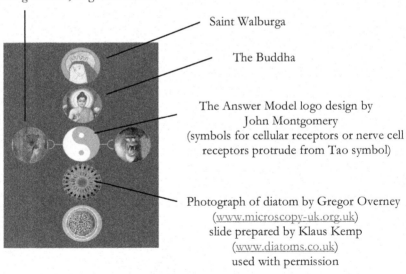

Saint Walburga

The Buddha

The Answer Model logo design by
John Montgomery
(symbols for cellular receptors or nerve cell
receptors protrude from Tao symbol)

Photograph of diatom by Gregor Overney
(www.microscopy-uk.org.uk)
slide prepared by Klaus Kemp
(www.diatoms.co.uk)
used with permission

www.theanswermodel.com

CONTENTS

INTRODUCTION

This is a book about addiction and how to overcome it. But addiction, as you will see throughout this book, is hardly confined to drug addicts, alcoholics, or compulsive gamblers. It is deeply embedded in the behavior of nearly everyone who lives in the modern world. Addictions are like parasites that sneak into the most powerful circuits in the brain – those that govern our basic survival instincts – and, by hijacking those circuits and manipulating their core biochemistry, profoundly influence, and even dictate, our thoughts and behavior.

Many people think addiction means being unable to resist something that provides overwhelming pleasure. But in this book we will suggest almost exactly the opposite: being addicted means being unconsciously attached to, unconsciously driven towards, pain and distress. In our view, the simplest types of addictions are the so-called "neuroses," in which people become stuck in loops of negative emotion like obsessive anxiety or worry. The reason, we suggest, that "neurotic" people become stuck in loops of negative emotion is that they are literally *addicted* to those emotions. The reason so many of us find it so difficult to change self-destructive and self-defeating patterns is that these patterns are *addictions*. The brain receives a similar, although typically less intense, biochemical reward from worrying as it does from drugs like cocaine or methamphetamine, and the habit is similarly difficult to break.

Like all addictions, an "emotional" addiction to worry or anxiety is driven primarily by the stress, or "fight-or-flight," response. Any heightened emotional state or experience of stress will activate such a response and trigger the release of stress hormones. Researchers have found that stress hormones such as cortisol have effects in the brain that are almost identical to the effects of addictive drugs like cocaine. And since stress triggers the release of hormones that have very similar effects to addictive drugs, it follows that anything we perceive as being stressful, including anything that creates emotional pain, can potentially become addictive.

5

Consciously, most of us believe that we do our best to *avoid* anything stressful, painful, or unpleasant, and this is probably very often the case. But all of us know someone who seems to do quite the opposite – perhaps unwittingly, they seem to do what they can to make themselves miserable. They worry excessively even though worrying never helps their situation; they become extremely anxious about something relatively unimportant; they consistently get into relationships that everyone knows will only bring them pain; and when they encounter something likely to bring them a measure of joy or happiness, they find a way to sabotage it. This kind of behavior is, of course, far easier to detect in others than in ourselves. But the perhaps disconcerting reality is that almost all of us do some version of the same thing. We often have clever justifications for even our most self-defeating habits, but to a clear-eyed observer, or an astute psycho-therapist, it couldn't be more obvious that most of us engineer painful situations and create pain within ourselves for no good reason. There seems to be a driving force underlying that part of ourselves that reason does not easily appeal to. And that force, we are suggesting, is biochemical addiction.

Any heightened emotional state, whether pleasant or unpleasant, can potentially become addictive. No such state is *intrinsically* addictive. But because these states all produce chemicals that are rewarding to the brain, they are all *prone* to addiction, and any of us can potentially succumb to such addictions if we are emotionally or physically out of balance. Occasionally recalling a painful romantic affair that ended ten years ago, for instance, could well be part of healthy emotional processing. But to re-engage those memories and relive that pain several times a day for days or weeks or months at a time almost certainly indicates addiction – it's the unconscious brain's subtle way of creating an emotionally-stimulating thought just to get a biochemi-cal reward, or "drug payoff."

We also believe that addiction is wholly responsible for what psychologists and philosophers have long called the "false self." The false self is the self that we believe ourselves to be, or think we need to be; but, in reality, it is merely an inauthentic veil that covers and disguises the True Self, the only authentic source of love, aliveness, and wholeness. The ultimate goal of all psychotherapy, and of all emotional, psychological, and spiritual healing, as the psychologist Carl

Jung said, is the dissolution of the false self and the discovery of the True Self.

The model we will present suggests that a person's false self is the collective expression, the sum total, of his or her specific addictions. We refer to the false self as the "addiction persona." We believe that addictive behaviors are connected to one another in an associative neural network within the brain, and that this linkage explains why one type of addictive pattern – such as an emotional addiction to anxiety – often triggers the expression of another type of addictive pattern – such as the abuse of alcohol. Because of these associations, the addiction persona acts as a recognizable and distinct entity, or "self," that becomes manifested as the false self. The True Self, we further suggest, is the self without addictions.

In our view, the True Self is an expression of the ancient biological drive to achieve and maintain balance, or homeostasis. Human beings experience homeostasis as a feeling of peace or well-being, or as a sense of emotional and physical balance. The drive to homeostasis, which is a fundamental principle in biology, is probably the most powerful force in all living things. In simple organisms, the homeostatic drive acts at a cellular level to automatically restore the proper balance of minerals and nutrients within each cell. But in humans, the homeostatic drive also involves complex emotional states and the *decisions* that those states influence and inform. The True Self, we suggest, is the force that maintains homeostasis both at these higher emotional levels, and also at the lower cellular levels.

All addictions, we believe, dysfunctionally drive a person away from biochemical and psychological balance. When people act out of the True Self, therefore, they make decisions that tend to bring them *into* psychological and physical balance, or homeostasis; and when people act out of the false self, or the addiction persona, they make decisions that tend to drive them *out* of balance.

All types of addiction – whether they are emotional, behavioral, or substance addictions – can be identified and resolved using our system. Because our approach deals directly, we believe, with the root cause of all psychological dysfunction, the process is both shorter and more transformative than traditional psychotherapy. And since all addictions, including drug addiction, have the same fundamental dynamics, overcoming one addiction makes it far easier to overcome others. As each addiction is resolved using our method, as each person becomes more and more conscious of dysfunctional drives that were previously unconscious, the structure of the false self is further weakened.

Our view of addiction is very similar to what Buddhists call "attachment." Buddhists similarly believe that anyone who can overcome his or her attachments will achieve enlightenment, the equivalent of living out of the True Self. But despite its undeniable power, the Buddhist path to enlightenment often seems mysterious and opaque, and many people, perhaps Westerners in particular, seem to have great difficulty in truly following that path. Carl Jung, for example, believed that Buddhism is essentially inaccessible to Westerners, that most Westerners simply do not have the cultural or historical frame of reference to appreciate Buddhism at a deep level.

Our own method for overcoming addictions – or attachments – is highly accessible to Westerners, and indeed is founded on Western science. Thus our method, in addition to being a novel form of psychotherapy, also represents a new path to spiritual enlightenment. Our approach contains many elements of the Buddhist sensibility, but merges that sensibility with Western neuroscience and psychology. The model we will describe therefore uses biochemical addiction as a connecting point not only between classical psychology and modern neuroscience, but also between Western science and Eastern spirituality.

The first six chapters of this book provide a solid foundation in the theoretical basis for The Answer Model. Since our book *The Answer Model Theory* explains the scientific underpinnings of the model in detail, our goal in the current book is to present only the science that is necessary for understanding and benefiting from the healing method. These first chapters show how addictions of all types operate by sending people inappropriately and dysfunctionally into various states of "survival mode." Addiction, in other words, sends us into survival mode when our survival is not particularly at risk. The dynamic begins as an over-protective, hair-trigger impulse to defend our survival against threats. But because of the substantial biochemical rewards that survival-mode states always supply, such states can easily begin to exert a dysfunctional, magnetic pull on us.

We will also present a detailed model that we believe explains the vast majority of the "mind-body" effects that have long been known to psychotherapists, and that have recently been receiving more attention from neuroscientists. We'll show that when the mind is thrown into a survival-mode state as a consequence of the addictive drive, the *body* will also be thrown into survival mode in various respects. We believe that this addiction-driven triggering of the body into different versions of survival mode explains, directly or indirectly, the great majority of physical illnesses in modern life.

Chapters 7-10 describe higher-level effects of addiction. We'll discuss, for example, how addictive dynamics often cause us to choose romantic partners who supply us with dysfunctional biochemical payoffs that result from relationship "dramas." We'll also talk about dysfunctional belief systems, one of the most all-embracing forms of addiction.

Chapters 11 and 12 will discuss the critical role of intervention in overcoming addiction, and the role of internal and external triggers in activating dysfunctional neural networks in our brains. These networks can be interrupted and ultimately broken down by the use of what we call "neural antibodies." Because addiction is fundamentally irrational, it always relies on illusions and lies for its sustenance. Neural antibodies primarily act to reinforce the *truth* about our circumstances and how we respond to those circumstances. Once you've built effective and stable neural antibodies, they will protect you from addiction and help break down the neural networks that have been perpetuating addiction in your life. As these dysfunctional networks begin to weaken, they can be replaced by healthier, more functional networks.

Chapter 13 shows how addiction corrupts dreaming and various types of play. Chapters 14 and 15, the final chapters of the book, connect our model of addiction, and the basic biological principle of homeostasis, to the highest spiritual pursuits, principles, and experiences. We'll show how the homeostatic drive creates a clear path for achieving spiritual enlightenment. We'll also suggest that the drive to homeostasis represents a powerful force that has been alluded to in all the major spiritual and religious traditions. Finally, we'll see how the principle of homeostasis, when combined with the knowledge of how the addiction persona and the True Self operate, creates an inexorable momentum towards homeostasis for all of us.

Addictive behavior is not something biological evolution prepared us for. It is rather a consequence of unnatural circumstances that have, for the most part, existed only since the invention of agriculture about twelve thousand years ago, when our ancestors began to leave behind the hunter-gatherer lifestyles that human beings are most naturally adapted for. These new circumstances, and the dysfunctional, addictive drives they have given rise to, have thrown most people badly out of balance. Only consciousness of how addiction operates, we believe, can bring modern men and women, and ultimately modern life itself, back *into* balance. In this book we will try to give you that consciousness, so that, if you wish to, you can overcome your own addictive patterns. If you want to hang on to some of your addictions, that's always something you can choose. Just be aware that, despite appearances, despite the illusion, when you choose addiction, you're always choosing pain.

In a real sense, addictions are never consciously "chosen" at all, but are rather fallen into unconsciously, or at best half-consciously. Whenever we compulsively behave in ways that are unnecessarily destructive to ourselves and to others, we always do so out of addiction. *Addiction* is what imprisons us, and addiction is what we need to be liberated from if we are to be truly free.

CHAPTER 1

PAIN, PLEASURE, AND SURVIVAL MODE

Human beings, like all living things, are built for survival. Our hunter-gatherer ancestors were sculpted and engineered by evolution to serve one overriding purpose: surviving and reproducing so that their genes could be successfully passed on to their offspring. The genes we carry within the cells of our own brains and bodies were left to us by those ancestors, and if those hunter-gatherers had lacked that all-embracing focus on survival, they themselves would not have survived and reproduced, and their genes would not be the ones we would be carrying today.

The will to survive permeates every aspect of the brain's normal operation. When our survival is particularly at risk, our brains shift, often dramatically, into high-alert, hyper-aroused states of what could be called "survival mode." The most overt state of survival mode is a sense of fear, or terror, that may be triggered, for instance, when we're directly threatened with physical attack or annihilation. But many other more subtle states of survival mode are equally common and important. As we'll see in the next chapter, strong sexual desire often becomes a state of survival mode. So does the emotion of anger, or the feeling of being somehow "less than" other people, a particularly common feeling in modern life that is a critical driving force in most addictions.

Hunger for food is often also a state of survival mode. If we don't eat, of course we won't survive. The feeling of hunger creates an intense, pervasive drive to find food, and the drive becomes more and more insistent as the nutrients in our bodies and brains are used up without being replenished. Once the state or feeling of hunger has driven us to find food and satisfy that burning need for nourishment, we're biologically driven, like all other animals, to settle back into a more peaceful, balanced state called homeostasis. After a hungry domestic cat has eaten, for example, it will often happily wash itself and then stretch its body out comfortably, perhaps on the couch, with a blissful and beatific look on its face. This is a cat in homeostasis. Since it feels no pressing needs and senses no imminent threats, there is no need to be in a state of survival mode. You may never guess it from the way many people live, but we human beings also evolved, at least in general, to be in a stressed-out, hyper-alert state only when to be in such a state is critical for our survival.

Addictions of all types occur when the brain gets tricked into thinking that there is a survival emergency when no such emergency exists. Addictive drugs like cocaine and methamphetamine actually create many of their effects in the brain by triggering a massive stress response and creating a powerful, although usually unconscious, state of survival mode. Similarly, when you're under the spell of a non-substance addiction, or of any type of behavioral or emotional "drug," you get thrown into a survival-mode state like anxiety for no compelling or objectively persuasive reason. The longer you remain in the state of survival mode, the more the part of the brain that drives this impulse is hesitant to allow you to leave the state because then, it believes, you will be in even more danger. An additional force that tends to draw you back in the survival-mode state, and often keep you there, is the substantial biochemical rewards that such states supply, as we'll see in more detail later. All forms of addiction, whether they are emotional, behavioral, or substance addictions, keep the brain and body in a nearly perpetual state of survival mode – the polar opposite of the more peaceful, balanced state of homeostasis.

One hallmark of the survival-mode states that all addictions utilize is the activation of a stress, or "fight-or-flight," response. The stress response is evolutionarily extremely ancient, and is almost identical in all mammals, reptiles, amphibians, and fish. Two of the main products of the stress response, adrenaline and cortisol, prepare the body and brain for "fight or flight" by, among other effects, increasing blood pressure and widening arteries so that enough blood can flow to the major muscle groups that are critical in any emergency response. The terms "fight or flight" and "stress," however, are highly misleading labels for this response. Sexual desire, for example, activates all the components of the so-called "stress" response – but sexual desire is hardly what we would typically think of as an emergency or "fight-or-flight" situation.

The stress response could more appropriately be called the "survival" response, because it apparently evolved to be activated under circumstances that are critical to our *survival*. The reason sexual desire activates the stress response is that such desire is critical for reproduction, which, in an evolutionary sense, amounts to *genetic* survival – the survival of the genes that our offspring are vehicles for. As is the case for any organism, our foremost biological objective is to pass our genes on to the next generation. The stress response is triggered whenever our brains decide that our survival or reproductive prospects demand that we *act*.

Two other brain chemicals that are released as part of the stress response are beta-endorphin and dopamine. Many studies have shown that beta-endorphin is the primary pleasure chemical in the brain – that is, when beta-endorphin is released into our brains, we often experience a feeling of pleasure or euphoria. Although it was long thought that *dopamine* was the main pleasure chemical in the brain – a claim that is still often heard – the evidence is now overwhelming that this is not, in fact, the case. Instead, what dopamine appears to do is create a "drive state" in the brain that motivates us to move towards whatever we need for survival, such as food. When we crave or desire anything, dopamine release in the brain appears, at least in large part, to create that feeling of desire – a feeling that will often lead to action geared towards pursuing or acquiring the object of desire. But when delectable food, for example, is found and then actually *eaten*, the pleasure and satisfaction that we feel from eating arises from the release of endorphin in the brain.

Why would endorphin, the primary pleasure chemical in the brain, be released as part of the stress response? At first this seems to make no sense. When the stress response is activated, it often indicates that we're fearing for our lives or are otherwise severely stressed, rather than feeling pleasure. But the apparent reason that endorphins evolved to be part of the stress response is that endorphins, in addition to being pleasure chemicals, are also potent analgesics, or *pain-killers*. Endorphins are opiates that are very closely related chemically to morphine and codeine, and are therefore very handy to have around in an emergency.

Whenever we think about our own evolution, about why our brains and bodies are built the way they are, we always need to remember that for millions of years humans and pre-humans evolved exclusively as hunter-gatherers, surviving only by hunting animals and gathering wild foods, such as fruits, vegetables, roots, and nuts. It was only when agriculture and animal husbandry methods were invented and began to spread about twelve thousand years ago that any other lifestyle became possible for us. And although there has been some evolution in the past twelve thousand years – such as the spread of a genetic mutation that allowed people to digest milk as adults – all of the known genetic changes that have appeared during this time appear to have been relatively minor and superficial. So our brains and bodies are almost exclusively designed for a hunter-gatherer lifestyle, although only a tiny percentage of human beings still live, in scattered pockets of the world, as hunter-gatherers.

For a wild animal – or human hunter-gatherer – any physical injury usually represents a true survival threat. Any animal with an injury in the wild becomes highly vulnerable to attack from predators, for example. Endorphins apparently evolved as part of the stress response because they kill the pain from a wound so that the sensation of pain won't be a distraction during an emergency. So if one of our hunter-gatherer ancestors were, for instance, attacked by a mountain lion, his primary goal and concern would be to either fight the animal off or escape so that he could survive. Feeling the intense pain from a serious wound would make it far more difficult for him to focus on fighting or escaping to safety. Once the emergency was over, however, and he was no longer under threat, the stress response would subside, endorphin levels would decrease, and he would finally begin to feel the pain from his injury. Then he would be driven to tend to his wounds in whatever way he could.

If endorphin is released during a stress response and is also the brain's primary pleasure chemical, why don't we feel pleasure when we're anxious, in pain, or otherwise severely stressed? There are likely to be a number of reasons for this. But the main explanation is probably that, even though we may not exactly derive a feeling of "pleasure" from the stress response, we do indeed appear to derive a reward from the endorphin release that is part of the stress response, although the reward is primarily unconscious.

What we always need to keep in mind about the brain's "pleasure center," or reward system – the neural system that provides us

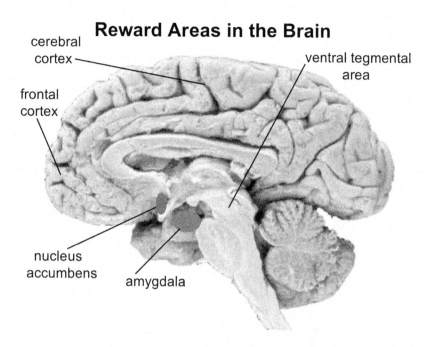

Figure 1: Two of the key reward areas in the brain are the nucleus accumbens and the ventral tegmental area.

with a feeling of reward, or pleasure — is that the core of it lies in a deep, primitive region of the brain. The primary components of the reward system are two regions, called the nucleus accumbens and the ventral tegmental area. They are buried like two large seeds beneath the cerebral cortex, which covers the brain like a thick, folded sheet (Figure 1). Neuroscientists refer to brain areas lying beneath the cortex as being "subcortical." Because the cerebral cortex is the seat of consciousness, or awareness, whenever we're conscious or aware of certain perceptions, thoughts, or actions, this consciousness generally arises from activity in the cerebral cortex. Anything that happens *subcortically*, or beneath the cortex, on the other hand, seems to almost always be unconscious — it occurs outside of our awareness. If the "pleasure centers" are being activated and rewarded, and they then in turn signal areas in the cerebral cortex about the reward, we may become conscious of the reward and experience a feeling of pleasure. But if the core reward areas don't send a signal to the higher brain regions in the cerebral cortex, we may remain entirely unconscious that we've received a reward at all.

Studies have shown, for example, that people who have drinks that are secretly laced with small amounts of methamphetamine, often strongly prefer this drink to another similar drink without the methamphetamine. But these people are usually entirely unconscious of the rewarding effects they are receiving from the drug-laced drink. In other words, because these people preferentially seek out this particular drink, they are clearly deriving some sort of reward from the methamphetamine, but at the same time they are not conscious or aware that they are receiving such a reward. We believe that whenever a stress response is activated, people similarly receive a reward from the dopamine and endorphin that are released as part of the response, but that they are typically unconscious or unaware of the reward. Furthermore, we believe that many people unconsciously seek out the biochemical rewards that stressful states will always supply.

Even calling these reward areas "pleasure centers" turns out to be highly misleading. Reward areas in the brain began to be called "pleasure centers" partly because brain imaging studies showed that these areas are activated by various pleasurable activities. When we eat, laugh, have sex, stare at beautiful faces, listen to good music, or are given money, for instance, a number of reward areas in the brain become strongly activated (Figure 2).

But researchers have also found more recently that these same reward areas – the so-called "pleasure centers" – are also activated during various *painful and distressing* states (Figure 3). One brain imaging study, for example, showed that sustained pain in a jaw muscle activates various reward areas and also triggers the release of substantial amounts of endorphin in these areas. Burns and electric shocks produce increases in endorphin in reward areas that can be comparable to receiving a high dose of morphine. It has also been known for at least two decades that large amounts of endorphin are released into the brain and body when self-mutilating "cutters" cut themselves.

Furthermore, it isn't only physical pain or distress that triggers a stress response and endorphin release in reward areas, but also *emotional* pain and distress. Emotional pain and physical pain actually create very similar responses in the brain, and various studies have

Pleasurable States and the Reward System

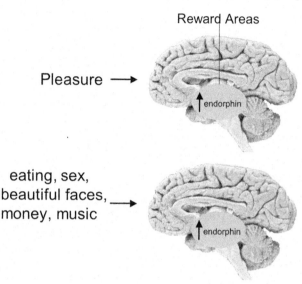

Figure 2: Brain imaging studies have shown that various pleasurable activities and behaviors — such as eating, having sex, looking at beautiful faces, receiving money, and listening to especially pleasing music — activate reward areas in the brain and release beta-endorphin.

shown that the experience of emotional pain, just like the experience of physical pain, activates reward areas and triggers the release of endorphins into the brain. When people with severe depression are told to think of an emotionally painful thought, for example, the thought itself can release large quantities of endorphin into their brains. When war veterans with post-traumatic stress disorder are shown films with reenactments of war scenes that trigger their own war traumas, many of them have powerful emotional responses – clearly representing survival-mode states – that release endorphin at very high levels.

Dopamine, the neurotransmitter of desire or craving, is also released during a stress response, probably for at least two reasons. Although dopamine creates a "drive state" in the brain that compels

Painful States and the Reward System

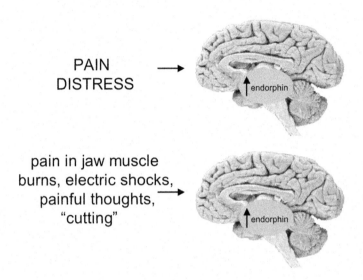

Figure 3: Many brain imaging studies have also shown that various types of pain and distress also activate reward areas in the brain and release endorphins. Examples include: sustained pain in a jaw muscle, burns, electric shocks, painful thoughts from the past, and mutilating or "cutting" oneself.

us to move towards food, for example, it also provides a drive state that compels us to move *away* from danger – such as a prowling mountain lion. Dopamine also plays a critical role in initiating the muscle movements that are pivotal in any emergency response. Enormous amounts of dopamine are released into reward areas of the brain during survival-mode states like anxiety. In the most extreme cases, the dopamine levels triggered by anxiety can be equivalent to the amounts of dopamine released after taking powerful stimulants such as methamphetamine.

Dopamine and endorphin, in addition to being released by painful or stressful states, are also thought to be the two most important neurochemicals involved in drug addiction and alcoholism. Addictive drugs dramatically raise dopamine levels in the brain – often to about ten times their normal levels – and also typically trigger a substantial release of endorphins, especially during the first few uses of the drug. Like painful and distressing states, addictive drugs throw the brain, in effect, into survival mode. And so pain, distress, and addictive drugs all release dopamine and endorphin into the brain as a consequence of states of survival mode.

If the dopamine and endorphin levels in our brains decline below a certain point, we feel terrible. We may lack the motivation to eat. We may lose our sex drive or even have trouble getting up out of bed. These brain chemicals, however, can not only be derived from survival-mode states, but also from healthy, homeostatic states – from sensual touch, physical exercise, healthy social connection, or from making love, eating healthy food, or simply being fully and vitally alive. But many people still find themselves repeatedly slipping into painful, stressful non-homeostatic states and getting their dopamine and endorphin payoffs by self-abusively lingering in those states. It's almost as if some people make an unconscious decision that being happy and fulfilled is an option that simply is not available to them – they won't be able to have fulfilling relationships, or a healthy, satisfying life in general, and so they will have to get their payoffs from pain, distress, and misery.

We can therefore get our dopamine and endorphin payoffs in two general ways: either from states of homeostasis or states of survival mode. Payoffs that arise from homeostasis and payoffs that arise from states of survival mode affect the brain very differently, however. When we're receiving "drug" payoffs from any state of survival mode, we become out of balance. The brain's biochemistry spikes past the normal, balanced state, and then will inevitably drop, or crash, far beneath that balanced state sometime later. Being in homeostasis never leads to such a rebound. Deep meditation, for example, which is probably the purest state of homeostasis we have access to, will never cause a rebound effect in the brain.

You could think of the difference between healthy payoffs and "drug" payoffs as being comparable to eating a balanced, complete meal, perhaps lean protein with some fruits and vegetables, and sitting down at the table and eating a handful of chocolate bars. In both cases you're eating and receiving biochemical rewards from the act of eating.

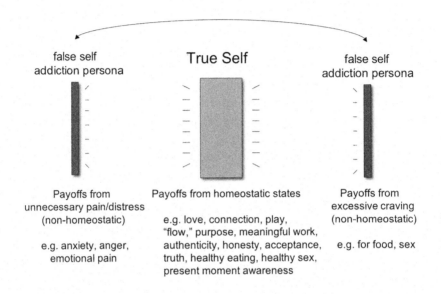

Figure 4: The human psyche is pulled in opposing directions by two "magnetic" forces: one arising from the True Self, which supplies healthy payoffs from various homeostatic states; and another arising from the false self, which supplies unhealthy, or "drug," payoffs from out-of-balance states such as excessive craving, anxiety, anger, or emotional pain.

But in the latter case, the chocolate and sugar will cause various aspects of your brain's biochemistry to spike and become distinctly out of balance. All addictive payoffs are like that. They cause your brain's biochemistry to surge, and that creates an imbalance that will keep you swaying back and forth on a pendulum – a boom and then a bust, a spike and then a crash. Healthy, homeostatic payoffs, on the other hand, will help keep you in a relatively steady, balanced state – physically, biochemically, and emotionally.

We believe that the only reason physically or emotionally self-destructive behaviors exist at all is that they supply a covert biochemical reward, primarily in the form of endorphin. In any behavioral, psychological, or emotional dysfunction, out-of-balance, survival-mode states such as anxiety or emotional pain are *used* – just like a drug – to derive a biochemical payoff. Thus nearly all psychological dysfunctions in human beings are ultimately due to the somewhat perverse fact that endorphin is released not only when we feel pleasure, but also when we experience pain.

The human psyche is thus typically fractured by two primary "pulls," or magnetic forces (Figure 4). The central force comes from what we call the True Self, which can be seen as the center of the psyche. The magnetic pull from the True Self arises because of payoffs that are released by healthy, homeostatic states, such as love, emotional connection, healthy eating, or healthy sex. These are states in which we are clearly *not* in survival mode – we don't feel our survival to be at risk and are enjoying ourselves, receiving copious amounts of healthy endorphin payoffs. The opposing force – which arises from the false self, or the addiction persona – provides biochemical payoffs from non-homeostatic, out-of-balance, survival-mode states, such as unnecessary pain or anxiety.

The competing payoffs from the false self and the True Self create a split in the psyche. While the false self, the addiction persona, unconsciously pursues survival-mode states to derive unhealthy "drug" payoffs, the True Self pursues pleasurable, homeostatic, *non*-survival-mode states to derive *healthy* biochemical payoffs. The biochemical payoffs released by survival-mode states ultimately underlie, we believe, nearly all unnecessary human misery and suffering. All addiction, all dysfunction, comes from compulsively deriving biochemical payoffs from painful, distressing, out-of-balance states. In the chapters that follow, we'll show how the false self, or addiction persona, is constructed by using these basic building blocks of addiction.

CHAPTER 2

FOOD, SEX, AND CRAVING

While it may be a challenge to see how anxiety or worry could possibly be rewarding, everyone knows that eating and having sex can make us feel very good. And there's really no reason why eating and sex shouldn't be completely pleasurable, why they can't be almost entirely free of conflict, guilt, or regret. But primarily because of the highly unnatural conditions that surround food and sex in modern life, many people relate to them in ways that are out of balance and, in our terminology, clearly addictive.

Pornography, for example, is something we are simply not well-equipped biologically to deal with. Nothing in our evolutionary heritage prepares us for the barrage and potpourri of highly stimulating images, often specifically catered to our own unique tastes and desires, that pornography presents us with. Hence it's very easy for pornography to throw some people out of balance – to lead them to spend hours watching it, at the expense of the rest of their lives, and then to either regret that lost time, or feel shame about it, or have it drive them into poor decisions with real-life sexual partners.

Addiction operates in two main ways. It derives biochemical payoffs simply by creating or perpetuating inherently unpleasant, distressing states, such as anxiety, and then generating dysfunctional payoffs directly from those states. It also, however, takes activities or behaviors that are inherently *pleasant,* that could otherwise be almost entirely pleasurable, and *contaminates* them by introducing unnecessary pain, distress, and states of survival mode. This latter dynamic is what happens in any food or sex addiction.

The key step in food and sex addiction is compulsive craving or desire. Various studies have shown that the feeling of craving – just the *thought* of craving something or someone – triggers, just like an addictive drug, the release of both dopamine and beta-endorphin in the brain. So the feeling of craving can potentially be *used,* although typically unconsciously, to derive a drug payoff. Engaging in a sexual fantasy, for instance – just the act of creating arousing images in one's imagination – will generate significant biochemical payoffs. Instead of taking a hit from a crack pipe, you can work yourself into a frenzied state of craving and just let the self-generated endorphin payoffs percolate through your brain.

A sex addict, for example, will get an extended drug payoff from obsessing, often for hours or days, about a particular fantasy. But the vast majority of the time, the actual sex act, whatever it might be, will be a disappointment. When any of us persist in obsessing about some intense desire, sexual or otherwise, we need to somehow *justify* the obsession, and typically that justification involves over-valuation of the object of desire. Consequently, if and when we attain that desired object, it will inevitably fall short of the illusion we've created to justify the craving. Part of the reason this pattern is so common is that if extended craving is the lead-in to any act, the craving for the act will almost always provide more drug payoffs than the act itself. In a similar sense, the anticipation artfully created in a Hitchcock movie will generate more tension and drama, and release more adrenaline in the viewer, than just showing the murder and moving on to another scene. Many substance abusers will tell you that the highest high they experience is often the high they get *before* they take their drug. It's the craving, the drama, imagining the buy, planning the buy, going to the buy spot, that often provides the biggest drug hit.

An intense craving or obsession sends a signal to the brain that you really *need* something, and when you need or want something that badly, the unconscious mind interprets the object of your desire as a survival need. Consequently, any intense craving will throw us into survival mode. If a hunter-gatherer is obsessed about something, it will usually be about something critical to survival, such as a game animal that he or she needs as food. But in the modern world, we may, for example, meet a potential romantic partner and begin to think about that person obsessively. When we obsess about someone in this way, usually it's because this particular person throws us into some sort of survival-mode state – they disconnect us, remind us of early dysfunctional relationships, early traumas, they trigger some strong *need* in us, make us feel vulnerable and "less than." We *need* them and their attention – we *have* to have it or we're going to *die!* That's the message that obsession sends to the brain's survival centers. And the brain responds by throwing us into survival mode.

The compulsive nature of this kind of obsession, as with all addiction, comes about because the state of survival mode has such a strong magnetic pull. It keeps pulling us back, as if our survival really were at risk, and as if the continual emergency situation required our complete, obsessive focus and attention. When the dynamic reaches its most fevered and dysfunctional pitch, we allow ourselves to be inappropriately thrown into survival mode for one primary reason: to receive the drug payoff that all survival-mode states supply.

Being obsessed with a potential romantic partner is not peaceful or even necessarily very pleasant, but it sure beats being depressed and hopeless. Obsession, however, like all addiction, only creates the *illusion* of vitality and aliveness. In all likelihood, we're obsessing about something that we're projecting onto the other person, something that isn't even *real* – we're obsessing about an *illusion*. That illusion further feeds the obsession and then the obsession requires the illusion to sustain itself. This is the hall of mirrors that every type of addiction draws us into.

Another truly insidious consequence of excessive craving is that it frequently leads us into very poor choices. These choices are "non-homeostatic" choices, in that they arise from a false state of survival mode and end up driving us even further out of balance, further away from homeostasis. After lingering in that state of craving for hours or days, we may end up making regrettable choices like eating a gallon of ice cream or sleeping with our best friend's spouse. Then after we commit the unfortunate act, we'll typically experience negative emotions like guilt, shame, and regret. Guilt, regret, and shame are all different versions of emotional pain, and emotional pain releases endorphin into the brain. Thus the dysfunctional, non-homeostatic, payoffs begin to multiply – not only do we get them from the excessive craving, but from the negative emotional states that we feel after we've made the poor decision that the excessive craving drove us to. This is the cycle of all addiction – swinging from one out-of-balance state to another.

Contrast the previous scenario with a healthier, more functional one. You meet someone you really like and are immediately attracted to. You get to know them, you talk about your lives and experiences and feelings, and begin to develop an authentic emotional connection, which adds to the physical attraction. You develop true feelings for this person, but you don't idealize them – you don't create unwarranted fantasies in your mind, you just stay connected to what you actually feel about them. At some point, one that feels just right, the two of you end up making love, and it feels great, it feels satisfying physically, emotionally, and spiritually. There is no regret, no shame, no guilt. The decision to have sex was well-considered, and it wasn't motivated by an over-driven craving artificially heightened by an illusory fantasy about the other person. This is a homeostatic relationship to sex – it is sex that is not driven by an artificial state of survival mode.

In a similar sense, there's also no reason that any of us should have any negative feelings about food and our relationship to it. In practice, of course, it can be very tricky. But we can have a purely homeostatic relationship to food, and to anything else, by simply being aware of how addictive dynamics operate.

Anorexia, for example, is essentially a chronic state of starvation, or physical hunger. Such a state of hunger will activate the stress response and trigger the release of dopamine and endorphin in the brain. In addition to chronic hunger, anorexics will almost always create a "drama" surrounding the decisions about whether or not they should eat, what they should eat, and about the fear of what they might look like after they eat. Any emotional "drama" will also stimulate the stress response and trigger the release of dopamine and endorphin in the brain. Thus the anorexic, like any other addict, or any other neurotic, becomes thrown further out of balance by continually deriving dysfunctional, non-homeostatic payoffs.

Binge eaters will typically marinate in their craving for particular foods for hours or even days. As with all addiction, part of the driving force is the presence of unnatural conditions we're not well-prepared for biologically. Such conditions can often trigger us into unhealthy patterns. In this case, the unnatural condition is the dizzying and alluring array of stimulating food items that are almost always available to us in modern life, and that frequently have unnatural effects on our biochemistry, sending us profoundly out of balance. But cravings for food are also often driven simply by an unconscious desire to receive a biochemical payoff from the *craving itself* – a desire to use the feeling of craving as a drug. At some point the excessive craving may throw you so far out of balance that you succumb to it – you eat the entire gallon of ice cream. Then you feel physically ill, ashamed, regretful – and receive more dysfunctional payoffs, and are thrown even further out of balance.

Not uncommonly a binge eater is also bulimic. The ride on the pendulum in this case would typically begin with uncontrolled, compulsive eating, which was probably prepared by hours of extreme craving. This manic bout of eating will be followed by purging – which is physically highly distressing and unbalancing – and then by the feelings of shame that will almost always accompany this pattern. At some point later, the shame will eventually shift back into an intense craving, which will lead to more uncontrolled eating, and the continuation of the cycle. This is the pendulum of non-homeostasis, the rhythm of all addiction. And the further any of us go into out-of-balance, survival-mode states, the harder it becomes to come back into a balanced state of homeostasis, so we can derive biochemical payoffs in healthy ways. Thus the addictive cycle is perpetuated.

Another version of this same boom and bust pattern – the exciting, overly-stimulating, and usually poorly-advised eating and sex that's often followed by regret and shame – is seen with chronic anxiety. Anxiety and depression are almost always co-morbid – that is, a person who suffers from chronic anxiety will also almost always suffer from chronic depression. A person with chronic anxiety is continually triggered into the survival-mode state of anxiety, usually for reasons that are not the slightest bit life-threatening. The state of anxiety then triggers the release of stress hormones that will provide a drug payoff to the brain. And the lingering state of anxiety itself will then continue to trick the brain into thinking that a true survival emergency really does exist. The perception by the brain that a state of emergency exists will therefore tend to reinforce the state of anxiety, thus delivering more drug payoffs, and thus perpetuating the whole cycle.

You may be worried, for example, that a large asteroid is at some point – some point very soon, perhaps – going to hit your neighborhood. And, who knows, you could be right. But is there any point in worrying about it? No. Still, the worry creates anxiety, which triggers a stress response and delivers a drug payoff. Now you're in a very anxious state, literally fearing for your survival and that of your family. Maybe this particular worry becomes too silly to worry about anymore. But, alas, there are plenty of other worries that can take its place, many of them with at least somewhat plausible justifications. Maybe your house will be destroyed by a fire. Maybe your children will be kidnapped. There's always something you could be anxious about.

The anxiety may cause you to act in ways that makes whatever you're anxious about less likely to happen – like clearing brush around your house to reduce the fire risk. That's a very functional response to the anxiety. But after you've cleared the brush, and taken other reasonable preventative actions, there's really no point in worrying anymore. What we're suggesting is that the underlying reason for the anxiety, in almost all cases, is simply the drive to get a hit of a drug. It's an unconscious way of putting your mouth on the crack pipe of anxiety and inhaling.

But no one can remain in a constant state of anxiety forever. Driving the stress system so intensely for long periods would begin to do enormous damage to both the brain and the body, and eventually would kill you. If meth addicts went on drug binges continuously and indefinitely, they wouldn't survive for very long. Maybe you've been almost continuously anxious for three weeks straight, using your false, and perhaps frankly absurd, justifications for all the anxiety you've been creating in your life. You've been getting the anxiety drug for three weeks. But at some point you have to stop.

And what happens when you stop? In effect, you withdraw the drug from your system, just like a substance abuser who temporarily stops using methamphetamine or cocaine. Your previously over-driven stress system will now suddenly be driven only moderately. But during the previous anxiety binge, your brain had adjusted to the drug being delivered at very high levels almost constantly. So when your anxiety levels finally begin to decrease, a form of "drug withdrawal" will set in. The symptoms of depression are actually almost identical to the symptoms of drug withdrawal, and the sudden withdrawal of any drug will typically trigger depression. We believe that in the great majority of cases, that's what depression amounts to – the consequence of withdrawing dysfunctional biochemical payoffs that have been released by states of survival mode.

This isn't to say, however, that you won't be receiving dysfunctional payoffs from the depressed state, because you will. One almost universal feature of depression is the almost constant reinforcement of emotionally painful thoughts. Depressed people are particularly prone to ruminating about painful events in the past, going over and over those events in their minds, obsessively recycling their feelings of shame, anger, and regret. And as we've seen, painful thoughts will produce biochemical payoffs, particularly endorphin, in the brain.

We believe that all psychological dysfunctions follow this same pattern. You're typically hoisted up onto one end of the pendulum of non-homeostasis (Figure 5) by using some sort of stimulant. It could be a literal drug stimulant, such as methamphetamine, or it could be anxiety or anger, or excessive craving for food or sex, which act operationally in the brain as "emotional" stimulants. When the stimulant, or "upper," is withdrawn, it will create a depressed state and lead to a swing to the other side of the pendulum. The dysfunctional payoffs from the depressed end of the pendulum are more comparable to "downers," or depressants, and are typically released from painful thoughts that are obsessively repeated and recycled. We believe that this same basic dysfunctional pattern drives all psychological dysfunctions.

How does addiction hold us in such a potent grip while it does such awful things to us? By playing on our survival instincts, by tricking us into thinking that our survival is at risk when it is not. Addiction holds a toy gun to our heads and we play along as if the gun were real. Then addiction can have its way with us. Once we're afraid, addiction can keep holding the button of our fear while it creates whatever illusion is necessary to allow it access to the drugs that it seeks.

Addiction is wily and it is cruel. But there's nothing *real* about it. Although addiction manifests as if it were a parasite, it is a parasite with no bodily form and no real intention. Addiction is a blind weaver of illusion, an unnatural pattern that tends to become activated when we're placed in circumstances that we're not biologically prepared for. Addiction can be visualized, for simplicity, as a separate self, or even as devil or demon. But in reality it is only a trick of the brain. It ultimately arises from a simple evolutionary quirk that at some point in

The Pendulum of Non-Homeostasis

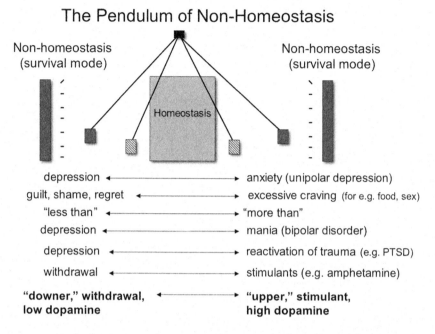

Figure 5: The pendulum of non-homeostasis suggests that a back-and-forth emotional and physiological pattern underlies all psychological dysfunctions. All the emotional states on the right side of the pendulum act as stimulants, or "uppers," and all the emotional states on the left side of the pendulum act as depressants, or "downers." When people are stuck on this pendulum, they swing from one out-of-balance, survival-mode state to another rather than remaining in homeostasis. This figure, for completeness, shows additional types of addictive patterns and conditions that will be discussed later in this book. These patterns are also discussed in more detail in The Answer Model Theory.

the distant past allowed endorphins to be released by pain. With the consciousness of how unnatural environments affect us, however, and with the knowledge of how the patterns that cause us so much pain are activated, we can overcome any addiction.

Whatever keeps us unnecessarily out of balance promotes addiction and dysfunction, and whatever keeps us in balance, in homeostasis, promotes health and well-being. It's really that simple. Does it sound boring to be "balanced" and "healthy"? It isn't. Being balanced provides *true* excitement, an excitement about being alive and about being connected to yourself, to the people you love, and to your true intentions in this world. An out-of-balance excitement is driven by a false intensity – it is exaggerated, "pushed," "claimed," just to get more adrenaline, more stress hormones, more drug. And when you push it too far in one direction, there will inevitably be a crash in the other direction. It's a basic law of the brain's biochemistry.

Any exaggerated intensity will activate an intense stress response, which will generate a lot of dopamine, for example. The brain responds to the increased dopamine by reducing the number of dopamine receptors, lest all the electricity generated by the pairing of dopamine with its receptor become toxic to the brain and potentially kill brain cells. Then, when the emotional intensity and stress response come back down, as they inevitably will – because anything too prolonged would be lethal – the dopamine levels will come down also. But the dopamine *receptor* levels will still be low from the excitement binge. So until the brain can adjust and make more dopamine receptors, there will be low amounts of dopamine transmission – low amounts of the activity generated by dopamine binding to its receptor. And that will mean low energy, listlessness, an unnaturally muted desire to live, to experience. It's an out-of-balance state on the other side of the pendulum, the depressed end, that necessarily must accompany the out-of-balance state on the other end, the manic or over-stimulated side. So this pattern is simply inescapable once the drug stimulant has been introduced.

Addiction hoists us onto that pendulum, and the ride always leads to more pain. Homeostasis is a smooth orbit, with plenty of excitement as well, but excitement that is *real*, that is organic, that comes out of and serves the wholeness of the self. When desire, for example, is authentic, when it's felt in the moment and is not exaggerated by an illusion, there's no reason to think that it's at all unhealthy. But addiction becomes disconnected in that it takes part of us and exaggerates it, stretches it, *uses* it to make us dizzy and disoriented. If you have a naturally high libido or sex drive, for example, the addiction persona will try to take that high libido and make a sex addiction out of it. The sex addiction will then take you on that pendulum, with the inevitable wild swings and the renewed, and often more intense, feeling of the "void," the emptiness, the deep hurt. A charge that is generated in such an unbalanced way will have a counter-charge, a swing back of the pendulum. The void is due to the disconnection that addiction feeds on and then consequently worsens. Addiction pulls you apart, it disconnects you from yourself.

On the other hand, picture an authentic, peak experience. You've trained for years as an athlete, or a musician, and during a competition or performance, you reach a state of "flow" where you're doing what you've been highly trained to do, and don't care what anyone thinks of you; you're just alive, in the moment, intensely and effortlessly focused on what you're doing. You have that exquisite feeling of joy and bliss and aliveness, of fulfilling all of your potential in that moment. You're serving a purpose, pursuing a passion, making a difference in other people's lives. Or you may feel a moment of deep connection with a romantic partner, or an intense moment of creativity, when you think of something original, or find a way to express something you've felt but have never been able to express before. Maybe you just have a random moment where you feel intensely alive and deeply at peace, deeply happy.

The True Self, which arises from the homeostatic drive, is naturally driven towards states of flow, towards purpose, meaning, connectedness, and present moment awareness. But if that drive is blocked or thwarted, the addictive drive tries to *mimic* it. Unlike addictive patterns, authentic states of flow typically have no negative repercussions at all. Quite the opposite. They not only create intense sensations in the moment, but also memories and experiences that will sustain you in the future, when you've fallen out of balance, when you don't feel so hopeful, peaceful, or vitally alive. They are connected to the deepest parts of you.

Heightened sensations that come from addictive patterns are *disconnected* – they take one aspect of your True Self and manipulate it, distort it. The more disconnected the emotions or sensations are from you as a whole, the more infested they will be with addiction. It can be desire, or some other artificial thrill, or it can be something painful – regret, guilt, or shame. Part of you really *does* have this desire, part of you really *does* feel regret or shame over something you've done. The addiction persona will isolate that part of you and distort it, manipulate it so that it can squeeze the drugs from it. But there will be a consequence to that artificially heightened state – a lowering of mood, a feeling of being lost. The pendulum will swing you back to where you were before, and it will swing through all of your emptiness, through that aching, hopeless void.

If you allow it to, the addiction persona will corrupt every aspect of your True Self by contaminating it with unnecessary survival-mode states. In its full dysfunctional bloom, addiction merely uses the True Self as a portal for drugs – it will do and use *anything* to get that drug payoff. Addiction will stuff anything into that crack pipe – any experience, any behavior, any aspiration, any emotion.

CHAPTER 3

"LESS THAN" AND ADDICTION

If there's one thing human beings detest, it's the feeling of being "below" another person, the feeling of being somehow "less than" someone else. All group-living animals have some sort of dominance hierarchy, or "pecking order," and no animal appears to enjoy having a low position in that hierarchy. But the feeling of having low status, in any real or imagined sense, seems to be especially stressful and distasteful for human beings.

The enormous disparities in wealth and status found in modern life have almost no parallel in our evolutionary history as hunter-gatherers. Before the invention of agriculture about twelve thousand years ago, such status differences – except in rare cases – simply did not exist. Because we evolved primarily to live in hunter-gatherer bands, which are remarkably egalitarian, we are simply not well-equipped biologically to have strong feelings of "less than."

A great deal of evidence suggests that people are far more prone to various psychological disorders when they feel they are "beneath" or "less than" other people. The reason for this, we suggest, is that the feeling of "less than" frequently triggers an unconscious emotional response that is due to our hunter-gatherer heritage. Specifically, when we feel "less than" in modern life, the feeling very frequently – either subtly or overtly – sends us into survival mode, a relic of our hunter-gatherer past when low status really *did* represent a significant survival risk, either in a genetic or an actual sense. And because the feeling of "less than" so often sends people into survival mode, this feeling or emotion acts as an important driving force for addictive behavior.

In most animal species, the consequences of having low status, particularly for males, can be profound. In monkeys, for example, the male animals who are lowest in the hierarchy are not only frequently bullied and beaten up, and not only have to scrap and struggle to get enough food, but they also have a very difficult time finding a female to mate with. While females of any rank are rarely at a loss for mating opportunities, the lowest-status male monkeys may never mate even once during their lifetimes.

Because their lives can be so difficult, low-status monkeys tend to release much higher levels of the stress hormone cortisol than higher-status monkeys. Researchers have also consistently found that low-status monkeys — when given the chance and supplied with the appropriate levers and feeding tubes — are far more likely to compulsively self-administer drugs than high-status animals are. The same is true in many other animals, including rats and baboons. Lower-status animals, in other words, are generally far more prone to becoming substance abusers, or drug addicts, than are higher-status animals.

Cortisol levels in humans are also influenced by status. One study of a college tennis team, for example, showed that the highest-seeded players — those with the highest "status" on the team — tended to have significantly lower levels of cortisol than the lowest-seeded players. And when formerly top-seeded players weren't playing so well and dropped into the lower seeds on their team, their cortisol levels tended to increase significantly.

People with the lowest socio-economic status not only have higher cortisol levels than those with higher socio-economic status, but are also, on average, far more prone to drug addiction and alcoholism. And these effects appear to begin at a very young age. Children as young as six years old who are from poorer homes have significantly higher cortisol levels than children from wealthier homes. These same children will also have a far greater chance of becoming substance abusers and alcoholics, on average, than children from wealthier homes.

Because stress hormones act in the brain in very similar ways to addictive drugs, it makes sense that the high cortisol levels triggered by low status would increase the risk for substance abuse. There are probably other, more complicated, reasons for the association between low status and substance abuse in humans, but the core reason, we suggest, is that having low status is very stressful. And people who are being chronically exposed to stress hormones are, in effect, already being chronically exposed to drugs.

Low socio-economic status is also very often internalized as low self-esteem, especially in young children. If a child has an ideal family situation, and receives caring and enlightened parenting so that his or her most critical physical and emotional needs are met, the psychological effects of low socio-economic status will probably be minimal in most cases. But, unfortunately, poverty typically acts as a terrible stressor for families, and a nurturing family environment is often extremely difficult to achieve and sustain under these circumstances. Feelings of low status in the parents, for example, are often unwittingly passed on to the children by, for instance, shaming the children or making them feel powerless or unimportant. If a parent is inattentive to a child's needs or frankly abusive, the child will very frequently, and almost always unconsciously, interpret that treatment as somehow reflecting his or her own self-worth.

Psychologists have long noticed a strong association between low self-esteem and neurotic behavior. Alfred Adler, for example, famously proposed that all neuroses are ultimately driven by an "inferiority complex," by a feeling of being somehow "below" other people. These feelings can very frequently have little or nothing to do with one's objective level of status, or with the extent of one's natural talents and gifts. It is clearly one's *subjective* assessment of where one places on some internalized hierarchy of worth that is most critical to self-esteem. Often a person's own assessment of his or her objective status level is wildly inaccurate, or frankly irrational. Victims of child abuse, for example, have notoriously low self-esteem. So do the substance abusers and alcoholics who, disproportionately, have either been abused as children or have grown up in severely dysfunctional family environments. Although family dysfunctions and low socio-economic status have little or nothing to do with the child who suffers through them, a child will very often develop low self-esteem by internalizing those dysfunctions and experiences.

The feelings of "less than," or low self-esteem, that are so endemic in modern life probably have a lot to do with misguided parenting methods and sensibilities, as we'll see in the next chapter. But they are also partly created by modern culture itself, which in many ways seems designed to *encourage* people to feel "less than." Advertisers, for example, are remarkably adept at making people feel "less than." To drive sales, advertisers often trigger a fear in us of being "less than," of not having enough, and then, in our state of fear and vulnerability, try to manipulate us into buying their products.

Our modern commercial culture is like a drug emporium. There are the overt drugs: the stimulants, depressants, and psychedelics – the wines, beers, and spirits, that wink at us from elegant, rainbow-colored bottles. Food is often presented pornographically – juicy, fatty meats smothered in oils and sauces, hundreds of ice cream flavors, chocolates of every conceivable variety that call to us from their shiny wrappers. Mixtures of sugars and salts are sprinkled, like a pheromonal musk, semi-secretly into nearly everything we eat and drink, causing our senses to race and spike unnaturally. Sexy models and celebrities excite our desire and envy, welcoming our illusory projections onto them with, as it were, open arms. Commercials use some of these models and celebrities, along with every other conceivable trick, every drug they can get away with using, to sell us a vast array of products that are usually, in truth, unnecessary at best. Addiction may be profoundly destructive, but it's typically very good for business.

The remarkable omnipresence of wealthy, sexy celebrities in the media can, among other things, very easily, and often insidiously, make the rest of us feel "less than." Indeed, celebrities often use the power of their images to endorse products that, if we can afford them, promise to bathe us in the magical aura of celebrity so that we can temporarily escape our feelings of "less than." If the product being peddled is purchased and then used or worn, surely we the consumers will feel at least a bit more like those models seem to feel. But the illusory projections onto these celebrities usually just further disconnect us from ourselves and from our own actual lives, and only end up reinforcing our sense of "less than."

To the untrained eye, many people with low self-esteem can come across as having healthy or high levels of self-esteem. This is typically because feelings of "less than" are often either concealed or compensated for with various unconscious strategies, such as arrogance or boastfulness, that aim to make such people both feel and appear to be "more than." Because the feeling of "less than" can often generate a driving ambition, people who are outwardly very successful are often found to be haunted by feelings of "less than." The healthiest ambition is driven by passion, by a love for what you're doing. Unhealthy ambition is driven by underlying feelings of "less than," and outward success is a compensation for those feelings.

Low self-esteem is always a companion of addiction – when you have one, you always have the other. And the lower your self-esteem, the more addiction you usually have. How can you tell if you or other people you know have low self-esteem? While there are no absolute, foolproof indicators, there are several warning signs, or red flags. Some of these are: people who brag about themselves a lot; people who usually keep their heads down or slouch, postures reminiscent of a submissive animal; emotional reactivity, such as having a volatile temper, or suddenly bursting into tears; and hyper-sensitivity to criticism or to perceived slights.

Another sign of "less than" is someone who has to be right, a "know-it-all." They're never wrong, they have to be right, because if they're not right, they'll be "less than," they wouldn't be "enough." Beneath needing to be right is always a pervasive feeling or fear of "less than." It's one thing to think that you're right about something and to defend the position strongly, as many people do. But when you *have* to be right, when you *need* to be right, that creates an imbalance; it becomes a fear of being wrong, which is really a fear of being "less than." *Needing* to be right, like any other strong need, throws us into survival mode, where addiction always does its work.

Most people who live in Western, industrialized cultures probably have at least a few of these "less than" qualities. But self-esteem levels are healthier in many other cultures. Hunter-gatherers, for example, at least before they are exposed to Western cultures, by all accounts have healthy and robust levels of self-confidence. The relatively minimal sense of "less than" in hunter-gatherer cultures supports one of our themes: that post-agricultural culture is primarily what drives people towards endemic feelings of "less than."

While only the most privileged people in industrialized cultures can afford certain kinds of luxury foods, for example, in hunter-gatherer bands, food is shared almost completely equally among the band's members. If any hunter in the group kills and captures game of any significant size, the meat will be scrupulously and laboriously divided into equitable portions to be shared with the rest of the band, and the triumphant hunter generally gets no more meat than anyone else, and sometimes will ask for no meat at all.

Power is also generally distributed relatively equally in hunter-gatherer bands. While there may be one or more individuals – typically older men – who are especially respected in the group, and who may acquire a certain kind of leadership role, their power is very limited. By nearly all accounts, all important decisions in hunter-gatherer bands, which usually consist of about twenty-five to fifty people, are made with the input and consent of most or all of the band's adult members. If any man with especially high status becomes imperious or arrogant, he will quickly lose the band's respect, and his influence will be greatly diminished. And despite the popular stereotype of Stone Age "cavemen" dominating and subjugating women, the status of women among hunter-gatherers is probably higher than it is in any other known culture. So our natural heritage, it turns out, is exceptionally democratic.

Since nearly all hunter-gatherers are nomadic or semi-nomadic, and since when they move to a new location they usually have to carry all that they own on their backs, they also tend to have very few material possessions. And so among hunter-gatherers, material things are rarely the basis for any status distinctions. For hundreds of thousands of years, at minimum, our human and pre-human ancestors pursued this lifestyle and operated within this relatively egalitarian social hierarchy. There is every reason to believe that this is the kind of social dynamic that our genes are optimally designed for.

But when agriculture and animal husbandry began to spread, beginning about twelve thousand years ago, this social dynamic changed dramatically. Hunter-gatherers need to be nomadic because, after several weeks or months in one location, they exhaust the food supply around their camp, and therefore need to move to a new site that will provide more game animals and plant foods. The development of agriculture, on the other hand, allowed groups of people to stay in one location for indefinite periods. More efficient methods of agriculture eventually provided a surplus of food, and the resulting free time and relative stability were often used to build permanent houses – rather than the temporary huts that nomadic hunter-gatherers typically live in – and accumulate possessions, such as pottery, baskets, masks, and decorative items like shell ornaments and feather plumes, that began to act as status symbols. In many cultures, the possession of livestock animals, such as pigs and goats, became a critical indicator of wealth, and greatly accentuated class and status distinctions.

Permanent settlements built on an agricultural surplus also soon became governed by leaders with infinitely more power than anyone could possibly achieve in a hunter-gatherer band. While all the men in hunter-gatherer bands were equally well-equipped with hunting tools that could also be used as weapons, the leaders of permanent settlements often had, in effect, a specialized military apparatus to support their claims to power. Among hunter-gatherers, small coalitions of men could easily overpower a band member who became too authoritarian. But in agriculturally-based settlements, the leaders and their supporters came to possess specialized weapons, techniques, and other critical resources that were exclusive to them. Their power, relative to the rest of the community, became enormous.

In the more developed agriculturally-based societies, such as the Aztec Empire in central Mexico during the 16th Century, the leaders often owned, at least in theory, all the land in their kingdoms, and had harems consisting of many hundreds of women. Slavery, which is unknown among hunter-gatherers, became widespread. The chasm between the ruler of the kingdom, who was often treated as a god, and the slaves, who were typically regarded as sub-human animals, would be utterly alien to any hunter-gatherer, who would rarely, if ever, experience anything we could even call a "class" distinction.

Although modern industrialized cultures have no slaves or rulers with god-like powers, the status distinctions between the richest and poorest people are still vast. There are also significant distinctions in modern life between those who have a substantial amount of power and those who have almost no power. This is also probably a critical factor in mental health – because feelings of powerlessness, just like feelings of "less than," can easily throw people into survival mode.

But although hunter-gatherer bands are exceptionally egalitarian compared to modern cultures, clear status distinctions do exist within each band. And the evolutionary stakes in the status game, particularly for men, can be extremely high. The highest-status hunter-gatherer men – typically the best hunters and the spiritual healers, or shamans – tend not only to attract the most desirable women, but often also have two or more wives. While any hunter-gatherer woman, generally without exception, can find a man to couple with, whether in a monogamous or polygamous setting, men who have the lowest status not only have the worst chance of attracting the most desirable women, but – especially if their status is *very* low – may not be able to find a woman to couple with at all. In an evolutionary sense, this is disastrous – it is genetic death.

Although modern people sometimes, often quite happily, opt not to have children, very few healthy people have no desire to have sex. Natural selection has genetically programmed us with the will to reproduce not, in many cases, by giving us a conscious desire to have children, but more discretely and covertly – by creating a strong sexual drive that very frequently results, particularly in the absence of modern birth control, in the presence of children.

Another danger of being a low-status hunter-gatherer is that low status can dramatically increase the chances of being abandoned by, or thrown out of, the band. If a man is an exceptionally good hunter, for example, his position in the band is probably quite secure, because meat is so valuable and necessary for hunter-gatherers to live and thrive. Similarly, any woman who is well-liked by other members of the band, and is also a productive gatherer, will probably also have a secure place in the band. But if a man, for example, is an inept hunter and *also* happens not to be particularly well-liked, his position in the band may be very tenuous. He may find himself in a very perilous situation if food supplies become low, and the band realizes that shedding a member or two may significantly increase the survival chances for the rest of the band. In this case, having very low status clearly represents an actual survival risk. Because if a band member is tossed out of the band, and is not able to join another band, he or she will be alone in the wilderness, and will almost certainly die.

In modern life, the typical consequences of low status are, fortunately, not quite so extreme. It's almost never a bad thing to have good looks, or a lot of money or education, and the relatively high status those attributes usually confer. But having or lacking one or more of these qualities is almost never a life-or-death proposition, especially in industrialized counties with strong safety nets and universal health care. There is usually some statistical reality to the fear that a drop in status will be a survival risk. When that risk is significant, it makes some sense to become distressed, but only if that distress motivates corrective or preventative action.

In a similar sense, anxiety is functional, in general, if it helps us to make good decisions with a level of urgency that's appropriate to the situation. If you're on a hike and see that you're being stalked by a mountain lion, it makes sense to become anxious or afraid – the adrenaline rush that accompanies the fear will probably help you to escape the danger and survive. If you're threatened with foreclosure on your house, the feeling of anxiety may motivate you to work harder, or lead you to make better decisions with your money. But once you commit to working hard and making good decisions, being anxious won't help you. In fact, quite the opposite. Overly high stress levels may, for example, make it difficult for you to sleep, which will make you more tired during the day and thus less able to work as hard as you might like to.

If it doesn't make any rational sense, in most cases, to become overly anxious and stressed about our jobs and financial status, why do so many of us do just that? There are two main reasons. First, the circumstances of modern life are so radically different from what we're best prepared for biologically that it's very easy for us to lose perspective on those circumstances. When most people are threatened with a relatively moderate drop in status, for example, they typically over-react in ways that are simply not appropriate to the situation. Second, because the survival-mode state of fear will always supply the brain with a drug payoff, biochemical addiction keeps pulling us back to the state of fear that is triggered by a threatened drop in status.

Biologically, a survival-mode state should only be activated when a true survival risk, or opportunity relevant to survival, exists. A woman sitting in a comfortable home, for example, with a husband and two children, who suddenly feels a suffocating feeling of "less than" after flipping through a fashion magazine full of sexy models, is not experiencing a true survival risk. She's being sent for a ride on the pendulum of non-homeostasis.

The trigger was reading that fashion magazine. Now, although, in actuality, men generally find this particular woman quite attractive, she feels fat, old, and poor. She starts thinking about that old boy-friend she had fifteen years ago, who broke up with her to be with another woman. She had felt so good about herself before that, so confident in her attractiveness, until *he* screwed it all up by hurting her so much. Her father, she's thinking, should really have complimented her more on her appearance. And if she had chosen a different profession, or married someone richer, maybe she could afford some cosmetic surgery – a little more here, a little less there. Then maybe she wouldn't feel so bad. Because the way things are going, her husband is probably going to leave her. What she really wants right now is fifteen or twenty chocolate brownies.

The specifics might be different in your case. But nearly all of us who live in the modern world go on that ride at different times in response to different triggers. Once you're triggered, once you go into survival mode, you get shuttled from one dysfunctional payoff to another. And each one of those negative thoughts, each one of those fears and self-induced pains, gives you a little drug payoff. The longer you stay on that ride, getting your drugs, the more out-of-balance and unconsciously hooked you become. You become so out-of-balance that it's very difficult to get out of survival mode and back to homeostasis, where you can start getting healthy payoffs again.

While the feeling of "less than" is one of the most common triggers that send us into survival mode, and into further addictive patterns, the feeling and state of "less than" can *itself* also become a strong addiction. A recent brain imaging study showed that when people experience a gain in status, reward areas in their brains become activated, presumably releasing endorphins. It makes evolutionary sense that gains in status would release endorphins and give us pleasure, because such gains are a boon to both genetic and actual survival, especially in hunter-gatherer life.

But the same study showed that a *loss* in status also activates reward areas, presumably also delivering an endorphin payoff. Healthy, functional payoffs are much better than payoffs from pain and distress – they almost certainly deliver more endorphins, and have the added virtue of not being associated with pain or distress. But a loss in status still does appear to provide a payoff. This probably happens for the same reason that other painful and distressing states provide a payoff: a loss of status, in the primordial hunter-gatherer environment, often represented a true survival risk, and so such a loss creates a state of survival mode that releases endorphins into the brain through the stress response.

Any psychotherapist is well-acquainted with people who seem to always be undermining or sabotaging themselves when something positive is happening in their lives. The secret or unconscious agenda of such people, we're suggesting, is driven by the dysfunctional payoff they get from their continued feelings of "less than." If they gave up the feeling of "less than" they would have to give up the drug they get from that feeling. As irrational and self-destructive as the dynamic is, that drug of "less than" keeps pulling them back, sending them for a ride on a pendulum.

In a broad sense, much of the unpleasantness in modern life boils down to people trying to be "more than" to compensate for their underlying fear of being "less than." But just as one tree is not "less than" another, one human being can't be judged as having more or less intrinsic worth than any other human being. Like trees, we are all different, we all have our own unique beauty and potential. Ranking people's intrinsic worth as "more than" or "less than" is an artificial, and even a violent, construct. There's a critical distinction between, on the one hand, making positive or negative *assessments* about people's behavior, and, on the other, overtly "judging" them. When we judge people in this sense, we in effect make them "less than" as human beings. And in making them "less than," we're making ourselves "more than." The whole dynamic is unbalancing and represents yet another back-and-forth pattern on the pendulum of non-homeostasis. Because although making other people "less than" by judging them makes us feel temporarily "more than," at some point we're going to judge ourselves also, and then we'll just swing back to feeling "less than" again.

The homeostatic approach to status is to see that while some people may have talents, qualities, or material assets that others lack, that doesn't in any way make their *intrinsic worth* greater or lesser than that of other people. People may do awful *things*, but that doesn't necessarily make them awful *people*. The most hardened criminal could wake up one day and start acting like Mother Theresa. But that person's intrinsic worth would presumably have stayed the same during the transformation.

We have a homeostatic approach to status when we see that no matter what assets we do or do not have, we are never "less than" anyone else as human beings. It simply isn't within our power or purview as fallible human beings to judge the intrinsic worth of another human being. When we ourselves can stop feeling "less than," we will have no conscious or unconscious desire to make *other people* feel "less than." Then we can finally become stable and secure in our own feelings of self-worth.

CHAPTER 4

PARENTING AND ADDICTION

The earliest periods in a baby's life are the most critical periods for the development of a healthy, homeostatic drive. For better or worse, human babies, like many infant mammals, rely completely on their caregivers to meet the needs that the homeostatic drive is designed to highlight and address. When babies are hungry or cold, for example, or aren't getting enough attention or love, they have a very limited repertoire of signals they can use to try to get those needs met. They can cry or express more subtle forms of distress with their faces and their bodies, and that's pretty much it. They can never *themselves* meet their needs – they can only send an alert to the caregiver, and then must rely on the caregiver, usually the mother, to respond to that alert and address those needs.

If babies are hungry, for example, that means that the state of hunger has driven them out of balance, into non-homeostasis. If the need is met promptly, the baby will quickly come back into homeostasis. The prompt recognition and meeting of needs promotes a healthy, homeostatic drive. But if a need is *not* met – if the baby spends extended periods in that state of need, and in the distress that results from not having the need met – the baby will linger in a survival-mode state like fear, anger, or hunger. And when people or infants linger for extended periods in survival-mode states, they become highly prone to becoming biochemically addicted to those states.

For babies in particular, the fear and distress caused by not having a basic need like hunger met promptly will activate an intense stress response. While the baby may, in reality, be in no danger at all, it will often interpret the situation as being an emergency, in which its very survival is in peril. The state of being in a perceived survival emergency, especially for an extended period, is so powerful – even for adults, and significantly more so for babies – that it tends to keep us in its grip. Any survival-mode state can also become reinforced because it delivers large amounts of dopamine and endorphin into the reward system. And the more time babies spend in non-homeostasis, in a perceived survival emergency, the more difficult it will be for them to feel safe and peaceful – that is, to be in a state of homeostasis. If babies can't derive healthy biochemical payoffs from being in homeostasis, they will consistently be driven into non-homeostatic states of survival mode and will receive more and more of their biochemical payoffs from the stress hormones that are released by such states.

Even in the womb, a baby, or fetus, responds very similarly to stress hormones and addictive drugs. The stress hormone cortisol is known to cross the placenta from the maternal to the fetal bloodstream, and so when maternal cortisol levels are high, the fetus will also be exposed to high levels of cortisol. When addictive drugs are taken by a pregnant mother, in both humans and animals, the drugs have been shown to have very similar effects on the fetus as high levels of maternal stress during pregnancy. In humans and many other animals, when fetuses who were exposed to either high maternal stress or maternal drug use become adults, they will, in both cases, have an increased risk of developing a disturbed stress response, various neuroses and psychopathologies, and substance abuse and alcoholism.

Stress and stress hormones, as researchers say, "cross-sensitize" with addictive drugs – that is, exposure to stress makes people more susceptible to addictive drugs, and exposure to addictive drugs makes people more susceptible to stress. The people who are most susceptible to neuroses, addictive behavior, and drug addiction are almost always those who respond to specific stressors with an especially intense stress response – their stress systems, that is, are especially "reactive," or "hyper-reactive."

Children who have been sexually or physically abused, for example, typically have stress systems that are strongly hyper-reactive, and this hyper-reactivity often lasts, to varying extents, into adulthood. Adult women who have been sexually abused as children have surges in their stress hormone levels in response to stressful situations like public speaking that are often several times higher than the stress hormone levels of non-abused women in similar situations. Abused children also have about a ten times greater chance of becoming substance abusers or alcoholics than non-abused children, and are at far greater risk for developing not only "neuroses," such as chronic depression and persistent anxiety, but also more serious "psychoses," such as schizophrenia.

More subtle aspects of parenting can also have profound effects on the stress response. Researchers who study "attachment" behavior can clearly test, for example, how bonded or "attached" children are to their mothers. Infants who are "securely" attached, who seem to have healthy, loving relationships with their mothers, generally have lower cortisol levels, and also have more moderate cortisol responses to potential stressors, such as being left alone temporarily with a stranger. Infants who are "insecurely" attached to their mothers have cortisol levels that are generally higher, and their cortisol responses to stressors tend to be both exaggerated and prolonged.

The influence of maternal care on addiction and the developing stress response seems to be extremely similar in all mammals. Experiments in rats, for example, have clearly shown how subtle aspects of maternal care can influence stress levels and the future risk of addiction in rat pups. Infant rats that are frequently licked and groomed by their mothers – that is, who receive higher levels of maternal care – tend to develop a moderate stress response and have a very low risk of becoming addicted to drugs when they become adults. But rat infants who are *less* frequently licked and groomed, who receive *lower* levels of maternal care, tend to develop a hyper-reactive stress response and are significantly *more* prone to becoming addicted to drugs. These infants are not being abused, mistreated, or unduly stressed – they are simply not receiving quite as much care from their mothers as the rats who are less prone to addiction. Although rats, of course, rear their young differently than humans do, these findings closely correspond to similar findings in a variety of other mammals, including humans.

The early influences of maternal care on the stress response clearly have lasting effects into adulthood – not only in rats, but in humans as well. Studies have shown, for example, that college students who have the most distant, least healthy relationships with their parents often become exceptionally nervous and have a dramatic stress response when giving public speeches or taking stressful math tests. In some cases, the stress levels of these students become so high that the amount of cortisol and dopamine released into their brains is equivalent to the amount that would be released if they took methamphetamine instead of a math test. But in the students who have closer and more loving relationships with their parents – those who seem to be more securely attached – cortisol and dopamine levels are often two to three times lower during public speeches or stressful tests. Other studies have shown that children who have more distant relationships with their parents are also far more prone to substance abuse.

The evidence that an overactive stress response in children is a critical risk factor for future substance abuse is overwhelming. But many studies have also shown that the development of an overactive stress system is a critical risk factor for various types of neuroses – or, in our terminology, emotional addictions. That is, people who have hyper-reactive stress systems are not only much more likely to become addicted to drugs or alcohol, but also to out-of-balance, survival-mode states like worry or anxiety.

Because emotional addiction and drug addiction both typically involve a hyper-reactive stress response, any circumstance or dynamic that increases the risk of developing emotional addictions will also increase the risk of developing drug addiction or alcoholism. And since addiction to survival-mode states like anxiety typically begins in early childhood, before drugs and alcohol are generally available, people's first addictions are almost always emotional addictions.

In the great majority of cases, therefore, the true "gateway" drugs are not addictive drugs themselves, but rather the stress hormones delivered by early emotional addictions to survival-mode states. When a baby's needs are not reliably met, the baby's fear and sense of unfulfilled need will repeatedly throw it into survival mode, and emotional addictions to fear, anxiety, anger and other states of distress will almost always be the result. These early emotional addictions will then set the stage for later, often more serious, addictions, such as substance abuse or alcoholism.

Hunter-gatherer infants and children don't seem to develop these types of emotional addictions. That may well be because hunter-gatherer parents are typically excellent at meeting their infants' basic needs. In nearly all hunter-gatherer groups, for example, infants receive round-the-clock, on-demand nursing for at least two or three years, and often for four years. Since hunter-gatherer infants are rarely apart from their mothers, whenever they are hungry, they generally have ready access to breast milk. This arrangement is ideal for the development of a healthy, homeostatic drive: whenever an infant is hungry, the necessary and perfect food is always available. Hunger sends the baby briefly out of homeostasis, but the constant availability of breast milk, along with the physical comfort of the mother's breast and body, brings the baby quickly back into homeostasis. There is no unnecessary emotional distress.

Hunter-gatherer mothers are also exceptionally skilled at "tuning in" to their infants and discerning what they need. Studies have shown that hunter-gatherer babies cry far less, on average, than American babies. Hunter-gatherer mothers also respond to their infants' cries far more readily and effectively, on average, than American mothers, and generally seem not only more attuned to the needs of their infants, but more attentive in addressing those needs.

Hunter-gather bands are filled with extended family who, according to nearly all reports, shower enormous amounts of love and attention upon babies born into the band. Most modern parents and babies aren't so lucky, frequently having more limited family support nearby, if they have any at all. So it often becomes impractical, or even impossible, for modern parents to supply their babies with typical hunter-gatherer levels of attention. And yet these levels of attention are presumably what babies are biologically wired to hope for and anticipate.

Although hunter-gatherers are generally excellent and attentive parents, life is often far from ideal. When the band is under great stress – from limited food resources due to a drought, for example – the infants in the band will inevitably get far less attention than when food is abundant. If things are *really* bad, and the adults in the band are themselves on the edge of survival, the infants in the band will become at significant risk for being neglected, or even abandoned and left to die by their parents. The awful reality of abandoning babies and children seems to be just as wrenching for a hunter-gatherer as it would be for any of us. But it's simply a matter of survival. Without such calculations and decisions, hunter-gatherer parents would never survive to have babies in the first place, much less take care of those babies after they are born.

Studies have also suggested that roughly one in every hundred babies born into a hunter-gatherer band, on average, will be killed soon after birth. Typically, infanticide occurs in one of two circumstances: either when the baby has a serious physical defect, which would dramatically lower its chances of surviving in the wild; or if the parents in the band are simply not in a position to support the baby. It is nearly impossible, for example, for a hunter-gatherer mother to nurse two infants at once – the drain on her energy, the demands imposed on her from carrying two infants around wherever she goes, and the need to give both of them nearly constant access to her breasts, simply makes the prospect impractical. Thus if a hunter-gatherer woman happens to give birth to twins, one of the infants, in most circumstances, will have to be killed. This isn't a matter of hunter-gatherers being callous or uncaring – they seem to be no more or less caring then we are. It is a matter of survival.

Babies have this evolutionary heritage wired deep in their brains. Their own survival depends on their being able to read cues in their environment so that their own chances of surviving are optimized. For all mammals, including human hunter-gatherers, abandonment and neglect are among the greatest risks for survival in the wild. The more attention an infant is getting, the better chance it has to survive, because more attention will almost always mean more care and more nurturing, more critical needs being met, and less chance of being abandoned. For babies, attention itself is therefore perceived as a survival need, much like food is. When babies aren't receiving enough attention, or when their needs are not being adequately attended to, they instinctively feel that their survival is at risk, that the risk of their being abandoned or severely neglected has risen to significant levels – thus they are almost always thrown into survival mode.

In most animals, including humans, the most critical factor that determines whether or not an infant will survive in the wild is usually maternal commitment to its well-being. In human hunter-gatherers, a strong commitment from the father is also pivotal for survival prospects. In the Aché hunter-gatherers of Paraguay, for example, the risk of a baby dying before the age of two goes up about four times if the baby's father dies. There's probably a comparable risk if the father abandons the infant and the infant's mother. Hence babies are always on the alert for signs of less-than-complete commitment from their parents. If they pick up signs that the attention they're receiving is inadequate for their needs, they will typically be triggered into survival mode. Although some parents interpret a baby in survival mode as being excessively demanding or controlling, this is to misunderstand how babies operate, and how they were designed by evolution. Babies just want to get their needs met, and want to feel safe and loved. If they're getting their needs met – substantial as those needs admittedly are – they will generally be quite pleasant, and their survival response will rarely be activated.

In most mammals, mothers that are anxious and inattentive are typically themselves struggling to survive. Any animal or human mother who is, for example, facing low and uncertain food supplies will generally pay far less attention to her infants and won't be as available to meet her infant's needs. Consequently, the stress, or survival, response of the infants will become activated. Strong activation of the stress response during infancy, many studies have shown, will modify behavioral patterns so that the infants become more anxious and fearful, or more aggressive. This makes sense biologically, because if there's a food shortage, things will tend to get nastier in every group of mammals, including humans. So it's adaptive for infants to be conditioned for the rough-and-tumble social dynamics they are likely to confront in these circumstances. That is, under difficult circumstances such as food shortages, being a little more wary or aggressive will promote survival.

One of the main themes in this book is that, in modern life, instinctual biological responses very frequently become corrupted by addiction, inevitably leading to dysfunctional behavior. And this is a perfect example. In hunter-gatherers, mothers only become anxious when *true* threats to survival, such as insufficient supplies of food, exist. The state of anxiety puts these mothers in a state of high alert that benefits their survival prospects under these circumstances. But in modern life, the chronic anxiety suffered by many mothers is primarily due to addiction. Significant threats to survival that require special attention rarely exist in modern, industrialized cultures. This isn't to say that lower-income people, for example, don't have a great deal of stress in their lives, and don't face true threats to their survival and well-being, because they obviously do. And, to a certain extent, temporarily higher stress levels may eventually lead to improvements in their well-being in some circumstances, and thus may occasionally be beneficial. But chronically high levels of stress are almost always maladaptive in modern life, for both wealthy and less affluent people.

So when people are chronically anxious in modern life, there's usually no *functional* reason for their anxiety. Indeed, chronic anxiety makes everyone *less* healthy. If a mother is anxious, for example, she will also almost always end up providing less care for her child. And this relative lack of care, as well as the effects of simply being around an anxious mother, will often create an anxiety addiction in the *child*.

It's almost impossible for people to be caring and attentive parents when they themselves spend most of their time in survival mode, lost inside an assortment of emotional addictions. When we're in survival mode, we instinctually become more self-absorbed and less nurturing. A chronic state of anxiety, especially when it is disconnected from actual circumstances, will distort all of our behaviors, including the way we parent.

The typical parenting pattern in modern life, although enormously variable, is in fact almost the exact opposite of the hunter-gatherer pattern. Too often, the core needs of an infant are not reliably met. One common ethos in modern parents, for example, is that their job is to somehow train their baby – in effect to control its behavior. Hunter-gatherers never seem to approach parenting in this way. They assume babies know what they themselves need, and their job as parents is to meet those needs. After hunter-gatherer children are weaned, they become increasingly independent and are encouraged to do things on their own, like hunt small animals or gather nuts and wild fruits. In modern life, older children are frequently overprotected, and often don't develop the sense of self-sufficiency that is so critical to the growth of healthy self-esteem.

Because hunter-gatherer parenting patterns are relatively uniform, and because they are the result of millions of years of evolution, we have to assume that these are the patterns that babies are biologically prepared to anticipate. Any significant variance from ideal hunter-gatherer parenting behavior could easily send a signal to infants that their circumstances may be truly dire, that they are experiencing a true threat to their survival.

Of course, modern life is very different from hunter-gatherer life, and the parenting methods of hunter-gatherers are often impractical in this new world, and perhaps not even optimal. And yet there's every reason to think that babies do best when those general hunter-gather parenting patterns are followed. If parents assume that babies typically send signals about what they need, for example, the parents can focus on "tuning in" to and meeting those needs. Infants who have their needs noticed and met will generally be happy and a joy to be around. They'll be living out of their homeostatic drive, on their way to realizing the full potential of their authentic selves.

But if an infant's needs are *not* met, it will be a very different story. In modern life, in the majority of cases those needs are not met largely because the parents or other caregivers are too disconnected from their *own* core needs, from their own authentic selves, to be able to be emotionally available for their children. People who are lost in their own addictive patterns simply cannot be good parents to their children. Consequently, babies will typically themselves become swept up in the addictive, non-homeostatic drive. They'll be spending so much time in out-of-balance, survival-mode states, because no one seems to see their distress, that they will become emotional addicts. They may be angry a lot, they may cry a lot, or they may shut down and hold their distress more inwardly by becoming very still and quiet.

Hunter-gatherer infants go into survival-mode states as well, but when they do so, it's because the threats to their survival are *real*. In hunter-gatherers, levels of parenting are generally consonant with actual circumstances. When circumstances are challenging, babies will often receive less attention, which will typically make them more anxious. But their anxiety, in this case, will be *functional*. Their level of anxiety will be appropriate to their circumstances and to the actual existing risks to their survival.

Particularly if a hunter-gatherer band is enjoying plentiful food supplies, however, a baby will almost always receive more than enough attention and love, and its needs will be rapidly and reliably attended to. Then the baby can just *be* – it doesn't have to *do* anything special to get attention, it can just be itself. This is how the True Self is nurtured, and how the healthy, homeostatic drive is established. But even under more challenging circumstances, the True Self will still be nurtured when behavior is tuned to *reality* – to circumstances as they actually are.

The genesis of dysfunctional "roles," which we'll talk more about in later chapters, probably begins as a consequence of early childhood dynamics that are unhealthy and dysfunctional. If an infant isn't receiving enough attention, for example, it will be thrown into survival mode because of the evolutionarily-ingrained associations that lack of attention will stir. Too little attention could mean impending abandonment; it certainly already means that needs are not being reliably met. Instead of just acting how it would naturally, the infant will then try to do things to get attention, perhaps to cry in a manipulative way, or do something especially "cute." When any of these behaviors are rewarded by attention, the baby may feel, quite literally, although unconsciously, that the behaviors may have saved its life. These "roles" then start to become ingrained, as does the pattern of believing that getting what one needs and wants requires playing a role of some sort, rather than just being whomever one is, and simply being authentic.

This is the beginning of the false self. The baby is jettisoning its authentic self because of a disconnection between its actual circumstances and the evolutionary dynamic that it is biologically wired to anticipate and respond to. The disconnection from the True Self has begun, as has a desperate need for attention that, from the child's perspective, seems survival-related and requires particular, often unconscious, strategies for its satisfaction. The disconnection will perpetuate a state of non-homeostasis, which will in turn almost always lead to a variety of emotional addictions.

CHAPTER 5

DISCONNECTION AND ADDICTION

Disconnection within babies or adults can take a myriad of forms, but one clear and especially common type of disconnection is a split between the mind and the body. People who have undergone severe trauma, such as repeated sexual abuse, can become extraordinarily disconnected from their bodily experience. Their legs, arms, or torsos may be in enormous pain or discomfort, their muscles may be as tense as violin strings, and yet they may be completely or largely unaware of it.

One very common response to trauma, whether subtle or severe, is to take very shallow, timid breaths and to freeze or deaden the body. This is an ancient biological survival response. Nearly all animals will do something similar when they feel their survival is at risk under certain circumstances. If a mouse moving around in its nest notices a cat walking by, for example, the mouse will freeze in place, barely breathing or moving, and hope that the cat will keep walking and not bother it. Freezing is a way that animals make themselves as inconspicuous and unthreatening as possible, hoping that other aggressive or predatory animals won't detect or harm them.

For humans too, the freezing response is sometimes perfectly natural and functional. If there's an angry bear nearby, quieting your breath, freezing in place, and laying low somewhere for a while may be exactly what saves your life. But in modern life, this freezing response is most commonly triggered by addiction. In modern circumstances, many people become anxious when there is no significant danger at all, partly because those circumstances are so unnatural, and partly because of an unconscious attachment to the drug payoffs that the state of anxiety will supply. Anxiety, a survival-mode emotional state mediated by activity in the brain, will then also unconsciously trigger or reinforce a physical survival response in the *body*. And a common physical manifestation of such a survival response is the freezing of the body. As we'll see in the next chapter, the phenomenon of an addiction-driven survival response in the brain triggering a comparable survival response in the body seems to explain nearly all the dysfunctional "mind-body" or "somatization" effects that can be so detrimental to physical health.

Inappropriate freezing of the body is due to a survival response being triggered when no real danger exists. The body of a former soldier with war trauma, for example, may become "frozen" with fear after he hears a car down the street backfire. The sudden fear will trigger a potent stress response, delivering significant biochemical payoffs to his brain, which will reinforce this particular case of post-traumatic stress disorder. In reality, however, there was never any danger at all, and both the emotional distress and the freezing of the body were unnecessary. The main driving force for the whole sequence was an unconscious addiction to the old trauma.

The freezing response can often serve another unconscious purpose. If a young girl is repeatedly sexually molested, for example, she may develop the habit of freezing her body, even when she's safe from her abuser, to dull the enormous emotional pain she feels from this gross violation of her physical and emotional integrity. Many studies have suggested that the brain, at least in large part, creates emotional states by interpreting changes in the state of the body. A drop or "pit" in the stomach that's triggered by an emotional injury like the loss of a loved person, for instance, at least partially creates the feeling of emotional pain. A racing heart is interpreted by the brain as fear, or excitement. The brain will then often send signals that sustain the elevated heart rate, thus reinforcing the emotion or state of fear. The body is the primary vehicle of emotion – when we're disconnected from, or not in tune with, our bodies, our emotions are deadened. So the habit of shallow breathing, because it makes us feel our bodies less, will often diminish the intensity of painful feelings such as those stirred by memories of sexual abuse.

This unconscious strategy of freezing the body to diminish painful feelings has some severe costs, however. First, it can easily conceal our own pain from conscious awareness, creating a disconnection between what we truly feel and what we are consciously aware of feeling. Any such disconnection within oneself – between the body, or feeling, for example, and the mind, or conscious awareness – will always be unbalancing. You can never be at peace, or in homeostasis, when you are disconnected from part of yourself, when different parts of you are not, in effect, speaking to each other. And because the state of disconnection that often follows traumas such as childhood abuse will tend to keep us out of balance, disconnection will always feed addiction.

In the present-day United States, levels of physical and sexual abuse in children are shockingly high. Careful studies have shown, for example, that roughly one-third of all girls in the U.S. have been sexually abused at some point during their childhoods.

But physical and sexual abuse of children is extremely rare in hunter-gatherers. Many writers and researchers have confused hunter-gatherer cultures, which have no agriculture, with other pre-industrial cultures that are agriculturally-based. These latter cultures often *do* have fairly high levels of physical abuse in their children. Parenting patterns have been shown to shift dramatically after agriculture is introduced into hunter-gatherer cultures, and these shifts seem to very frequently lead to an increase in the abuse of children. But any kind of physical or sexual abuse of children in hunter-gatherer bands seems, by nearly all accounts, to be extremely unusual. Since the hunter-gatherer lifestyle presumably reflects what we're best equipped for biologically, serious abuse of children is probably highly unnatural.

It is also probably extremely unnatural for any human infant to sleep apart from its mother, although the practice is very common in modern Western cultures. Hunter-gatherer infants never sleep apart from their mothers, and would categorically never sleep alone. An infant going to sleep alone at night in a typical hunter-gatherer hut in the wild would probably not be alive in the morning. Predators such as hyenas are acutely aware of vulnerabilities in their prey, and a lone human infant would be the easiest prey imaginable. Because of this evolutionary heritage, babies left alone at night in separate rooms will often shift into an instinctual state of survival mode. More subtle forms of trauma are also created when an infant's basic needs for food, love, and attention, for example, are not reliably met. These more subtle traumas, because they trigger survival-mode states, may also lead to a habitual freezing of, and therefore a disconnection from, the body.

Although habitual freezing of the body is often at least superficially effective in diminishing the intensity of painful emotions, it will also diminish the intensity of *positive* emotions, like joy, bliss, or excitement. Such positive emotions produce substantial biochemical payoffs in the brain. But any emotion – whether positive or negative – that is authentic, that is homeostatic, will release an endorphin reward in the brain that is completely healthy. When we effectively shut down our bodies, we get far fewer of these endorphin rewards. And we need that endorphin! We have to get it one way or another. If we can't get it in healthy ways, we're unconsciously driven to get it in *unhealthy* ways.

What are those unhealthy ways? They represent all forms of addiction. Addiction is when unhealthy, distressing, out-of-balance activities or emotions are unconsciously engaged in, or *used*, with the conscious or unconscious agenda of supplying biochemical payoffs to the brain. Because freezing or deadening the body will greatly diminish our ability to derive healthy biochemical payoffs, if we habitually freeze our bodies, we will almost inescapably resort to deriving unhealthy biochemical payoffs from addictive patterns as a compensation. It's one thing to freeze our bodies to protect ourselves from a bear attack. But if we spend most of our lives keeping our bodies relatively stiff or frozen – if we do it out of habit, as an established, unconscious pattern – we will almost inevitably become addicts. We will become emotional addicts, at minimum; probably also behavioral addicts; and perhaps substance abusers as well.

Hunter-gatherers, you probably won't be surprised to hear, seem to have a generally healthy relationship to their emotions. Many anthropologists have commented on how freely various hunter-gatherers express their emotions. In describing the Mbuti pygmies of central Africa, for example, the anthropologist Colin Turnbull noted how they tend to laugh so raucously that their laughter often develops into "near hysteria." Similarly, when the Mbuti are mourning the death of someone in the band, they mourn intensely, wailing and weeping, Turnbull wrote, "with what amounts almost to violence." But once the mourning period has passed, usually after a few days, everyone in the band is encouraged to go on with their lives, although the grief of some of the mourners will undoubtedly continue to linger. The songs the Mbuti traditionally sing at the end of this formal period of mourning reinforce an acceptance of the inevitability of death. But the songs are also, as Turnbull writes, "a sheer expression of joy in life."

This is probably an excellent general model for feeling and expressing emotions in a healthy, functional, way. If you just let yourself feel what you need to feel, you can pass through even the deepest grief. When you don't *use* feelings to get a drug payoff, those feelings won't linger for longer than they need to. You feel them, in their full, authentic intensity, for as long as you really need to feel them, and then you pass through them, you let them go. Then you can go on living. Even "negative" emotions, such as feelings of loss, or emotional distress, are healthy if they are *authentic* – that is, if they are not forced, not unconsciously manufactured or prolonged just to derive a biochemical payoff from them. We evolved to derive biochemical rewards from strong emotions. *We have to feel.* And if we keep ourselves from expressing and feeling those strong emotions, we'll unconsciously compensate by falling into a variety of addictive patterns.

An obsessive thought, for example, especially if it provokes fear or anxiety, triggers a stress response, and therefore provides substantial drug payoffs. Compulsive eating or compulsive sex do the same thing. When "cutters" mutilate themselves with razors or other sharp objects, this is simply another type of compensation, a more direct way that people can create pain within themselves to derive dysfunctional payoffs from that pain. But "cutting," like all addictive patterns, can also be seen as a dysfunctional way of trying to *feel* again. People who are consistently and chronically triggered into survival mode, and who become disconnected from their bodies, become incapable of deep and healthy feeling. But we have to feel, there is a deep and powerful drive within us – the homeostatic drive – that wants and needs us to feel. If our minds and bodies refuse to cooperate, refuse to be released from being in survival mode, that drive will become dysfunctional. The desire to feel will be filtered through addiction, and will therefore be expressed dysfunctionally.

All addictions work this way. They are dysfunctional attempts to recover the depth of feeling, the intensity that comes from a full experience of being alive. Addictions create experiences that are grossly distorted imitations of what it's like to be in a state of "flow." When we're *truly* in flow, we're completely engaged in what we're doing, whether we're playing a game, doing work we love, or just *being* and not caring what anyone else thinks or how they may or may not be viewing or judging us. But if we're not able to feel that intensity in a healthy, whole, and peaceful way, we'll soon become driven to feeling it in *unhealthy*, addictive ways: by out-of-control, obsessive sexual desire; by ravenous, compulsive, unconscious eating; or by unconsciously creating intense emotional pain and stress within ourselves. "If things cannot go straight," Carl Jung said, "they will have to go crooked." Addiction is what happens when things start to go crooked.

The disconnection within us that perpetuates addiction can also be seen as a reflection of the disconnection we face just by living in the modern world. Take the common modern experience of flying in an airplane, for example. Many people become highly distressed and anxious while flying in airplanes. Of course, being on a large commercial plane isn't as safe, statistically, as sitting comfortably in a house with smoke alarms and security gates. You're not *that* safe, but you're pretty safe. The danger is infinitesimal. And flying is a lot less dangerous than driving a car, as almost everyone knows. The main reason that flying can create so much fear and anxiety in so many people is that it's a very unnatural experience for us. We're simply not evolutionarily well-equipped for it. And it's the same with much of modern life – the unnaturalness of it creates disconnections and illusions that can easily fool us and lead us into dysfunctional behavior.

When you're flying in a plane and there's a fair amount of turbulence, the danger is minute, objectively it doesn't even register on any true danger scale. But it creates anxiety in many people because it's extremely unnatural for us to be suspended 35,000 feet above the earth and to have absolutely no control over our fate. And then even if there *is* a statistically significant survival risk – in a major winter storm, for instance – you're on the flight already, you've already made your choice. You're not piloting the plane and so it's out of your control. So what's the point of getting nervous? It really makes no sense.

But there are two primary factors that drive the dynamic. First, the situation is an unnatural one for which we're not biologically prepared. If we're being attacked by a mountain lion, how we respond *does* matter, and so having the fight-or-flight response is *functional*. But it isn't functional on a plane! Except in very rare emergencies, the stress response serves no purpose for passengers on a plane. By increasing stress levels, it actually *increases* our survival risk because it's *unnecessary* stress, which is unnecessarily detrimental to our health. The second factor is addiction – if we're not conscious of how addiction operates, we can start getting addicted to the anxiety and stress that can so easily be triggered by so many different aspects of modern life, including being inside a turbulent airplane.

Having no physical *control* over our circumstances is also very unnatural. Hunter-gatherers frequently climb trees, for example, to find delicacies such as honey from beehives that may be suspended high in the tree's branches. If you were a hunter-gatherer on a honey-finding mission in a tree, and the tree suddenly began to sway danger-ously, you would have a strong stress response. But the stress response would stimulate functional action – like climbing down from the tree! There are few, if any, circumstances in which a hunter-gatherer would not have a great deal of control over his or her physical circumstances. But when you're flying in a plane, you have *no* control. Aside from the event of an actual crash or other emergency, all you can really do is keep your seatbelt fastened, and that's about it. We're simply not well-equipped biologically to deal with that lack of control. It's a disconnec-tion between the unnaturalness of our modern circumstances and the biological responses that are instinctual for us.

Disconnection and addiction always go together. And although external circumstances like flying on an airplane may reinforce or worsen the disconnections within us, ultimately disconnection always amounts to our being disconnected from the True Self because we're operating out of the false self. Part of the authentic self of every nervous flyer, for instance, knows that it makes no rational sense for them to become so anxious about flying. They know at some level that their anxiety is only hurting them. This kind of disconnection repre-sents yet another vicious cycle – because the more disconnected you are, the further you are from the True Self, and so the fewer healthy payoffs you will get. And because you need to get those payoffs from *somewhere*, this will feed the non-homeostatic drive, disconnecting you further, and removing you further from the True Self. This is the cycle that is common to all addiction. Addiction is driven by disconnection and further feeds and worsens disconnection.

Feeling a "void," a dark, hopeless pit inside that can send you tumbling into unspeakably awful feelings of emptiness, similarly indicates that something inside you is disconnected. Some core need of yours is probably not being addressed, perhaps a need for love and emotional connection. Something is definitely askew. Maybe you're not facing something that you need to face. Maybe it's some old pain that you haven't let yourself feel, that you're disconnected from.

The thing about feelings is that, to be healthy, you need to feel them, you can't be disconnected from them. But you also don't want to get stuck in them. You don't want to keep putting them in your crack pipe just to get a drug payoff. Feelings are cheap, they're always in abundant supply. If you need a hit of something, you can always locate an emotion that delivers a nice dose of the drug you're craving. Surely there's some old pain you can re-engage, and you can marinate in that for a bit. And there *are* a lot of things you could worry about. What about all those people who screwed you over, who were so mean to you for no good reason – why not be angry about that? They deserve it, they *deserve* your anger! God knows they caused you enough pain. If it weren't for them, you'd be feeing a lot better right now.

You can have all the angry and painful thoughts you want, of course, but they won't dispel the "void," because the underlying need you have will still be unmet. You could have compulsive sex with a variety of different people, or you could voraciously devour whatever food seems appealing at the time. But the void will remain. Indeed, compulsive sex and eating will only widen the void, because they will create even more pain, and disconnect you even further from what you truly need.

Modern parenting, it must be said, very frequently begins the process of disconnecting children from themselves. This disconnection can be brought about in many ways, but the dynamic often includes both neglect of a child's true needs, and some sort of controlling, over-indulgent, or over-protective approach to parenting the child. Under this kind of parenting, many children never get a sense of self. They don't have any ownership over their lives; they don't really make their own decisions or choices, but are instead manipulated into making decisions and choices that are driven more by the parent than the child. So they flounder around in a lost state, ripe for a variety of addictive behaviors. Ultimately, however, they are only "lost" because they are disconnected from the True Self. There's a disconnection between who they think they are and who they really are – between what they presume to feel and what they really do feel.

The distinction between healthy and unhealthy feeling is, at least in theory, a clean one. Healthy, functional, feelings are those that simply pour out of us in the process of being alive. Unhealthy, dysfunctional feelings are those that are called upon inauthentically and *used* just to get a drug payoff. In practice, however, making this distinction can be a lot trickier. We have to allow ourselves to feel, but then it's usually a good idea to try to determine whether the particular feelings we have could possibly be coming from addiction. Distinguishing authentic and inauthentic feelings often requires connecting both to the feeling state itself and also to our more rational faculties. But it also has to be experiential, instinctual – part of you just knows, senses, when you or someone else is being authentic, and you simply need to access this innate sense.

True authenticity is always very moving, it's unmistakable. Certainly, you can feel it, you *know* it, when someone is being *in*authentic. There are probably scores of signals that your brain and body pick up on, mainly at an unconscious level, that tell you when someone is being less than forthright, shading the truth, forcing their emotions just for effect. We all have a built-in system that detects and responds to authenticity and inauthenticity. But most of us need to get much better at detecting inauthenticity within *ourselves*. If you want to overcome addiction, if you want to commit to the homeostatic drive, you have to commit to authenticity, and you have to get better and better at detecting inauthenticity, especially within yourself. Because inauthenticity is always disconnecting, it always feeds addiction.

Furthermore, there *are* some clear red flags for dysfunctional, addictive feelings. The trustiest red flag is simply whether you've been over the territory many times before. If you've revisited the same scenario over and over, of how your friend or lover disrespected or betrayed you, hurt you, if you've thought of it ten or twenty or a hundred times, you can be all but certain that you've developed an addiction to the anger and hurt that the memory triggers. When you again recall the particular anger-provoking scenario, your jaw will probably clench, your face will tighten as if to squeeze just a little more endorphin and dopamine out of all that pain and anger.

Anger is a universal part of the human emotional repertoire only because it does have a functional purpose sometimes – anger is often useful when, for example, we need to defend ourselves against attacks or threats to our physical or emotional well-being. But when we become angry for no functional reason, we are using our anger as a drug.

Being dishonest also creates disconnection within us. When we're dishonest with another person, part of us knows we're being dishonest, while another part of us is trying to pretend that we're actually being honest. When we act in ways that are clearly unfair or unethical – when we lie to people, cheat people, manipulate people, do unnecessary physical or emotional harm to people – that also creates a disconnection within us. Part of us knows that what we did wasn't ethical; and part of us tries to somehow justify what we did. It feels infinitely better just to act in ways that we know are honest and ethical, that correspond with our deepest core values as human beings. Then there's no disconnect. Then we're at peace about what we said and what we did.

When we're disconnected from our emotions, we can do things that make us feel badly, that clearly aren't good for us, and yet not be aware of just how badly we feel. Or we may have an initially authentic feeling, but then have the feeling become "pushed," exaggerated, so that it overwhelms our system and doesn't allow us to feel other feelings that may truly be authentic. A sex addict may become so overwhelmed with a craving for sex, for instance, and that craving may become so biochemically overpowering, that he may not be able to access other feelings like shame, emptiness, or emotional pain. Indeed, one of the unconscious functions of the craving is to try to cover up those negative feelings – and it often temporarily, although dysfunctionally, succeeds in doing so.

Any intense chemical stimulant like amphetamine, and any "emotional" stimulant like anger, craving, or anxiety, will at least partially cover up other underlying feelings and disconnections. Emotional stimulants will also release endorphin, which, if you're in pain, will probably alleviate the pain to some extent. But, of course, the pain will just come back at some point, probably with even more intensity. Because you haven't addressed the true source of your pain at all – you've just covered it up with a drug.

CHAPTER 6

MIND-BODY EFFECTS

The mind and the body are intimately connected, and in a real sense are not separate at all. Anything that affects the mind will also affect the body, mainly through the so-called "autonomic" nervous system, which unconsciously triggers various bodily responses that correspond to various brain states. And anything that affects the body will also affect the mind, since the brain contains elaborate maps that are constantly monitoring and responding to the state of the body.

We've discussed at length how addictive patterns hijack the survival instincts by creating unnecessary states of survival mode. When this happens, the mind is sent into survival mode for no good reason. Addictive dynamics will use any ruse to convince the brain that survival is at risk when survival is clearly *not* at risk, or at least not to any significant degree. While the homeostatic drive is trying to keep us in balance, the addictive drive is trying to throw us out of balance, into states that are simply different versions of survival mode.

When the mind goes into any state of survival mode, the *body* will also go into survival mode. The body in a functional state of survival mode will undergo specific changes that would help any wild animal or human hunter-gatherer to prosper or survive in different survival-related situations, such as a physical attack. In the wild, both the survival risks and the subsequent responses tend to be of short duration, since survival threats themselves are typically also of short duration. You'll usually either be killed or mortally wounded by such threats, or the threats will pass relatively quickly. The survival response is turned on, and then when the threat passes, it's turned back off. With addiction, however, the survival response is turned on *non*-functionally, *in*appropriately, and often chronically.

The simplest case is with anxiety, or fear. Wild animals and human hunter-gatherers generally only become anxious when they sense a true survival threat. The emotions of anxiety or fear, along with the bodily responses that go along with those emotions, help us to prepare for or confront those threats. For humans in particular, however, many more subtle social situations and social cues can also trigger states of survival mode. These responses are largely an evolutionary remnant of our hunter-gatherer days, when social dynamics could in many cases create true survival risks.

Social isolation, for example, which is so common in modern life, can easily trigger the primal fear of being excluded from the life-giving hunter-gatherer band. If such isolation were experienced within the context of a hunter-gatherer band, it would represent an extremely serious survival risk. Social exclusion would greatly increase the risk of being thrown out of the band, and so could literally result in your being left alone in the wilderness to die. In modern life, not being invited to a birthday party or a wedding that's important to you can be extremely painful, but very rarely will it be life-threatening.

Social isolation in modern life is well known to be a major risk factor for various neuroses and psychopathologies. But this risk, we're suggesting, is largely driven by the addictive loops that such isolation often triggers. The survival instincts become confused, in effect, and the misplaced survival fears drive addictive patterns. The effects are mild in many people, but in others, because of their genetic vulnerabilities or histories of childhood trauma, the effects can be profoundly damaging both psychologically and physically.

All animals that experience a survival threat will have a number of characteristic responses in their bodies in response to the survival-mode state triggered in the brains. We've listed seven general categories of such responses below. Since we believe these seven general effects, along with other unnatural elements of modern life, are ultimately responsible for the great majority of the physical ills that people currently suffer, we'll go through the effects one by one. For each category, we'll discuss why the response enhances survival in an emergency situation, and then we'll discuss some of the bodily ills that can result from chronic, addiction-driven activation of the response.

1. Disturbances in heart rate and blood pressure. Any survival emergency will usually increase heart rate and blood pressure, due to the release of stress hormones like adrenaline and cortisol, which help to prepare muscles for fight or flight. But when the stress system is activated chronically, it can lead to high blood pressure and various heart conditions like atherosclerosis.

Studies have shown that hunter-gatherers almost never develop high blood pressure. Furthermore, the blood pressure of hunter-gatherers does not significantly rise with age, even when they reach their sixties and seventies. This is probably due to three major factors: moderate activation of the stress response, high levels of physical activity, and a healthy diet. Hunter-gatherers, for example, have about five times less salt in their diet than the average American. The link between a high-salt diet and hypertension has been clearly established, as has a link between hypertension and stress.

2. Raised Shoulders. Nearly all animals raise their shoulders and scrunch their neck downwards when threatened with attack. The main reason for this response is that raising the shoulders protects the vulnerable neck area. When dogs, for example, kill another animal, they typically sink their teeth into the nape of their victim's neck and shake the animal until it dies. Big cats, such as leopards and jaguars, similarly often lunge for the neck when they attack humans. Raising the shoulders makes our necks a smaller target area for any predator or dangerous human. But in both animals and human hunter-gatherers, once the threat of physical attack subsides, the shoulders will relax and sink back to the lowered position that is most natural and healthy for them. Addictive patterns, because they create chronic states of survival mode, will often keep driving the shoulders upward.

As any yoga teacher will tell you, people with tense, raised shoulders are remarkably common in modern life. If you look at many people's shoulder placement, you'll see that their shoulders are very commonly tense, and that they often hold their shoulders in an unnaturally high position, almost literally "at their ears." They are unconsciously protecting their necks. Years of having their survival response consistently activated, usually for no good reason, have driven their shoulders upward. But how many people who go to yoga classes are under constant threat of physical attack, or even frequent passing threats? Very, very few. Their shoulders are tense because their minds and bodies are almost constantly in survival mode as a consequence of addiction. The whole sequence makes no rational sense – but addiction never makes any rational sense. Addiction is a trick of the mind. And when the mind is tricked, the body will also be tricked, because the mind largely controls the body.

Many of us also go into survival mode and raise our shoulders when we're being attacked *emotionally*. When we're being indignantly accused of some wrongdoing, for instance, our shoulders will often tighten and start to creep upwards. At first, this may not seem to make any biological sense, since the attack is only an emotional or psychological one, and poses no obvious threat to the neck area. But if you're a hunter-gatherer being angrily berated by another hunter-gatherer, the chances go up significantly that this other person may also begin to attack you *physically*. Hence millions of years of evolution made the determination that when we're being attacked emotionally, it's often a good idea for us to protect ourselves and our necks by raising our shoulders.

Chronically raising and tensing the shoulders, however, can be extremely damaging to the shoulder joint and to the areas surrounding the joint. The shoulder joint will be out of balance, unnaturally straining various muscles and tendons and setting the stage for more serious shoulder injuries. The principle of homeostasis not only applies to the whole of us, it applies to every part of us: every cell, every body part, every joint. When one part of the body is out of homeostasis, it can easily throw other parts of the body and the mind out of balance as well. Chronically raising the shoulders exemplifies this general principle, since it will often also create strains in neighboring muscles in the neck, back, and chest.

Many people say that shoulder problems are simply age-related. But this is only partially true. Without addiction-driven raising of the shoulders, the shoulders of older people would probably generally be quite healthy, if not quite as healthy and robust as those of younger people. The shoulders of younger people are certainly more resilient to the unnatural postures that addictive dynamics create. But without addiction, there would be dramatically fewer injuries and shoulder problems at *every* age.

3. Jaw tension. Tension in the jaw is also almost universally seen in animals under threat of attack. While a dog's jaws, for example, are loose and relaxed when the dog is feeling relaxed or playful, its jaws will become very tense if it's threatened with an attack by another dog.

For many animals, including humans, biting can inflict serious damage on an attacker. Tense jaws are jaws that are ready to bite.

Any dentist or voice teacher can tell you how common jaw tension is. TMJD (or temporomandibular joint disorder), which is due to chronic jaw tension, can result in severe pain and restricted movement in the jaw. "Grinding" the teeth, especially at night, both results from and further creates jaw tension, and can seriously damage teeth and gums. But how many people do you know who have fended off attackers by biting them? How many people do you know who are constantly threatened with physical attack? Probably not many. And so what sense does it make to be constantly readying the jaws to bite someone or something that may attack you? It doesn't really make any sense. But addiction never makes any sense.

These responses are all unconscious. They are patterns that typically begin early in childhood when we feel, and in actuality *are*, more vulnerable to attack. They are also biological responses that are a vestige of our hunter-gatherer days, and, more distantly, our animal ancestors. In hunter-gatherer life, physical fights may frequently involve biting, as fights often do even today. These instincts and bodily responses were functional in our human and animal ancestors, but in us, in modern life, they are most commonly used in the service of addiction. And like everything else that arises from addiction, they only cause us pain and throw us out of balance.

Jaw tension is often specifically associated with the feeling of anger, which is a distinct type of survival mode. Wild animals frequently become angry when they are attacked, for example, or threatened with attack, because the emotion of anger fuels the bodily responses that help fend off an attacker. If you're not being threatened, attacked, or otherwise seriously thwarted in some survival-related endeavor, it doesn't make much biological sense to be angry. Of course, we also become angry when we're threatened *emotionally*, or threatened with the loss of an attachment figure, like a friend, lover, or spouse. But in hunter-gatherers, such a social loss could ultimately result in a true survival threat, such as a significantly weaker social position within the band, which could have many survival and reproduction-related consequences. In modern life, such losses rarely represent significant threats to survival.

Hunter-gatherers may also be thrown into survival mode when

circumstances call for *them* to be the attackers. If a man's wife is threatening to leave with another man, for example, the bereaved and angry husband may be motivated to attack the other man. In this case, he will typically experience both anger and all the concomitant body responses that are typically triggered by the emotion of anger, including jaw tension.

4. Erratic breathing. When we go into survival mode, our breathing becomes agitated. Breathing can either become rapid – which oxygenates the muscles to prepare for fight or flight – or it can become shallow, which is part of a "freezing" response. The freezing response, as we saw in the last chapter, evolved to make animals and human hunter-gatherers less noticeable and threatening to predators or other potential attackers. More submissive animals may also become very still so as to be as unthreatening as possible towards a more dominant member of its own species.

For people in the modern world, an inappropriate or dysfunctional freezing response is particularly common. When many people, especially those who were traumatized as children, start to feel strong emotions, especially anxiety or fear, their bodies will freeze, and their breathing will become very shallow. The vast majority of people freeze their bodies for extended periods almost solely because of their emotional addictions. Survival-mode states in these cases are typically driven by "neurotic" fears, like the fear of being unfavorably judged by another person, that, in modern life, typically have little or no bearing on survival prospects.

Again, in a hunter-gatherer context, being unfavorably judged by other members of the band may lead to your eviction from the band and hence quite possibly to your death. It's never much fun even in modern life, of course, to be disliked or to have your behavior or beliefs unfavorably judged by other people. But only very rarely will this create a true survival risk for you. You'd almost always be better off not allowing yourself to be triggered into any form of survival mode in this situation, and just to continue to breathe normally and comfortably, connecting to your full bodily sensation and feeling of aliveness.

Breathing in a shallow manner for extended periods can have very damaging effects on the body. All the cells in our body require constant replenishment of oxygen, and chronic shallow breathing may result in too little oxygen being transported to those cells. This core dysfunction is likely to result in increased susceptibility to a wide range of physical and psychological ills. Because shallow breathing is associated with a state of anxiety, it will also tend to perpetuate the anxiety, which will, for example, increase blood pressure. So shallow breathing is part of yet another addictive loop. That's why becoming conscious of the tendency to take shallow breaths in certain anxiety-provoking circumstances can be so powerful – you can purposefully take long, steady, deep breaths that can, at least temporarily, help break the cycle. However, if the brain keeps going into survival mode because of addictive dynamics, it will keep sending the body into survival mode also. Ultimately, the only lasting way to break this cycle is to address it at its source, which is emotional addiction.

5. General muscle tension. When dogs, for example, are under threat, all of their muscles become tense, ready to be mobilized for fight or flight. It's the same with people. Chronic addiction-driven bodily tension can have very detrimental effects on joints, tendons, and ligaments, and can make various injuries, such as pulling muscles or tearing ligaments and tendons, far more likely.

6. Stomach disturbances. When animals are threatened with attack and their survival is at risk, a very typical response is to defecate. It's also a very common response in soldiers during intense combat. In a survival emergency, there's no energy available to digest food, so you might as well get rid of the ballast of undigested food and make yourself lighter so you can run or fight more efficiently.

Although in most cases you won't actually evacuate your bowels, at least not immediately, when you're in a survival-mode state, your body will almost certainly put less energy into digesting whatever food is in your stomach. While foregoing digestion can help an animal or person to survive during a true emergency, chronic, addiction-driven stomach disturbances can have ruinous effects on the digestive tract. Of all the organ systems in the body, the stomach is probably the most sensitive to emotional upset. Whenever we're physically or emotionally stressed, the stomach will be severely challenged. Inflammatory bowel disorder and ulcers, for example, are well known to be highly stress-related. As Robert Sapolsky, a Professor of Biology at Stanford Univesity, points out in his book *Why Zebras Don't Get Ulcers*, although ulcers are usually caused by the bacteria Helicobacter, only about 10% of people who are infected with the bacteria actually develop ulcers. One of the key factors that determines which of those people who are infected with the bacteria will actually get ulcers appears to be high stress levels. And those high stress levels, we're suggesting, are almost always driven by addiction.

7. Immune system disturbance. The immune system has a complicated response in survival emergencies. The immune system becomes more active during the first thirty minutes or so of a stress response, but then becomes *less* active than normal if the stressed state lasts for an hour or more. The system may have evolved this way because a stronger immune response would often be needed to prevent infections from wounds received during an attack. But if an attack or other emergency lasts for a long time, the animal is better off decreasing the intensity of the immune response and using that saved energy to deal directly with the emergency situation. The body only has so much energy, and in a survival emergency that energy has to be used very wisely.

This survival-mode effect on the immune system is probably the most far-reaching effect of addiction-driven stress. Paradoxically, chronic stress can both result in autoimmune disorders – in which the immune system becomes so overactive that it begins to attack our own tissues instead of invading bacteria and viruses – but also in chronic immuno-suppression, in which the immune system is *less* active than normal. Robert Sapolsky suggests that people may become especially prone to autoimmune disorders when they have repetitive, short-term stressors. Because the immune system becomes overactive during the first phase of the stress response, repeating that phase over and over ramps up the immune response so that it often becomes overactive and dysfunctional, as in autoimmune diseases. While autoimmune diseases like Lupus, Crohn's disease, and Type 1 Diabetes are relatively common in modern life, there's little or no evidence that they exist in hunter-gatherers. Autoimmune disorders seem to be extremely rare in the wild.

A suppressed immune system, which often results from repeated stress that lasts for longer periods, is probably also an enormous risk factor for various illnesses and diseases. Studies have shown conclusively that stress makes people far more susceptible to catching the common cold, and also makes people significantly more likely to develop full-blown AIDS after infection with the HIV virus. People with chronic stress are also significantly less likely to recover from bouts of cancer. And although the evidence is less conclusive, it seems very likely that chronic stress-related immunosuppression not only makes people more susceptible to bacterial and viral infections, but to cancer as well.

Bacterial infections, viral infections, and various cancers clearly can develop from factors that are independent of chronic stress. What the evidence strongly indicates, however, is that chronic stress significantly increases the risk that various infections, and probably cancers as well, will develop. Studies have shown that hunter-gatherers, even those who live to old age, have at least one hundred times less risk of developing cancer than we do. The increased risk is probably due to many factors – especially diet, exercise, stress levels, and perhaps environmental toxins. But rates of cancer, even those not due to smoking or drinking alcohol, are dramatically lower in our natural state as hunter-gatherers than they are in modern life.

These seven survival response-induced bodily changes, along with unnatural diets and unnaturally low levels of physical activity, probably account for the vast majority of disease and bodily illnesses found in modern life. Since all of these dynamics are profoundly influenced by addiction, we suggest that addictive dynamics are directly or indirectly responsible not only for all or nearly all psychological dysfunction, but for the great majority of *physical* ills and dysfunctions as well. Other aspects of modern life, such as a far greater prevalence of bacterial and viral pathogens when compared to hunter-gatherer life, also probably play a large role. But research on hunter-gatherers suggests that if we ate our natural diet – the hunter-gatherer diet – and had hunter-gatherer stress levels and lifestyle patterns, we would be dramatically, almost incalculably, healthier.

Emotional addiction, like all addiction, continually sends the mind and body into survival mode. Some emotions activate certain bodily responses more than others, however. Anger seems to be particularly associated with jaw clenching and elevated blood pressure, while emotional pain seems to be particularly associated with disturbances in the stomach and the immune system. Due to specific genetic vulnerabilities and specific histories of trauma, different people will be affected in different ways by addictive patterns and addiction-induced stress.

Emotional addiction may affect some people primarily in their stomachs. Other people with strong, resilient stomachs will ruin their teeth by grinding their jaws together. Some may have chronically tight, sore shoulders because they are continuously and unconsciously protecting their necks from an attack by lifting their shoulders. Others will become hypertensive or develop autoimmune disorders like Lupus or Type 1 Diabetes. Since emotional addiction lays the foundation for all other addictions, and since addiction over-drives the stress response in a way that is ruinous to the body, the vast majority of these bodily ills, we're suggesting, are ultimately due to emotional addictions.

When the mind goes into survival mode and consequently sends the body into survival mode, the body, just like the mind, will become out of balance. If this out-of-balance state continues, the body will inevitably develop aches, pain, and eventually more serious syndromes that will not only perpetuate non-homeostatic states, but will also supply dysfunctional payoffs due to pain- and stress-induced dopamine and endorphin release in the brain.

Thus addiction will spread, in effect, from the brain to the body. The body, like the brain, will be caught in the addictive drive. If the brain isn't in homeostasis, or isn't obeying the functional homeostatic drive, at some point the body won't be in homeostasis either. But the converse can also happen: the *body* can get out of balance, say from a muscle pull, and this can send the *mind* into non-homeostasis. When both the mind and body are in non-homeostasis, they'll often both become entwined in the addictive drive, which will reinforce the out-of-balance state.

Ideally, the body and the mind are like two partners in a healthy relationship. In all healthy relationships, the relationship itself helps both partners stay in homeostasis, or to come back into homeostasis when either partner becomes distressed or out of balance. But all *un*healthy relationships consistently drive both partners *out* of homeostasis. The same is true for the mind and the body. If the mind starts to become anxious about falling asteroids, the body can, in effect, say to the mind: "I don't know what you're so anxious about. I feel great. I want to *live* and not worry about things that will probably never happen." If the body pulls a muscle, the mind can in effect say to the body: "Don't worry, I'll take care of you, I'll ice that sore muscle, and soon you'll feel fine again and we'll be back in homeostasis."

When you've had a lingering physical injury or painful condition, you may find yourself unconsciously split about the condition and the pain. Part of you wholeheartedly wants all the pain to go away. You may despair that the pain is never going to leave, that you're never going to get better. No one can guarantee that you're wrong – none of us will live forever. The great likelihood, however, is that if you allow your body to heal itself, it will heal. But a lingering pain can throw any of us out of balance. So there may be some part of you – the dysfunctional part – that starts to become a little attached to that pain. When we were children and a tooth was about to fall out, who among us could resist the temptation to manipulate the tooth with our tongues so we could enjoy a brief thrill of pain?

We can start doing a similar thing with other injuries. If your shoulder has been sore for a while, instead of relaxing it, you may do things with it that cause more pain. Maybe you're just "testing" it. Or maybe there's part of you that's getting a drug out of the pain. Your pain *will*, in any case, release neurochemicals in the brain that are potentially rewarding – that's simply an inescapable part of the biochemistry of the brain and the stress response. The question is whether any part of you is *using* that pain by prolonging or intensifying it and then stuffing it into your crack pipe. At least consider the possibility.

If you have any lingering, chronic physical pain, the likelihood is that at least part of you has developed an addiction to that pain. Are you doing everything you possibly can to alleviate that pain, to heal the physical syndrome you're suffering from? If not, then part of you is seeking that pain out of addiction. If that weren't true, why wouldn't you be doing more to alleviate the pain? Laziness? But in that case laziness would just be another more subtle form of self-abuse, of the self-destructive behavior that is driven by addiction. We can be remarkably clever and inventive at creating excuses and justifications for our self-destructive patterns. But these patterns always come down to addiction, and the basic dynamic of addiction is always the same.

If you're in physical or emotional pain, if you feel isolated or disconnected and don't know how to deal with those feelings in a healthy way, you might walk down the street for a cocktail or a beer. But you could also reach for one of the many emotions that always seem to be hovering somewhere around you. If you could just release one of them into your brain and your body, you could be flooded with those intense, strangely rewarding chemicals.

Various doors, various thoughts and recollections, can be opened to let each of those emotions back inside you, with a little coaxing, a little seduction. You might sneak off when no one is looking and twist one of those doorknobs with a glazed look in your eyes. Then you'll feel the anger, the anxiety, that lingering old pain that's never far away – the sadness, the craving, the hunger, the drama. Just open one of those doors and it all comes flooding back, unsettling your stomach and your breathing, tensing the muscles in your jaw and in your shoulders. Soon you may start to feel the tightening again in your back or in your hip. Nerves will start to pinch, tendons and ligaments will tighten. Joints will be slightly askew, like faces that are squeezed and pulled in opposite directions. Maybe you'll inadvertently, or unconsciously, bump into your coffee table and wail at the throbbing pain. By allowing addiction into your brain and into your body, by granting it access to all of your pain, you've given it the power to create even more pain.

CHAPTER 7

ADDICTION "ALTERS" AND THE ADDICTION PERSONA

The addiction persona is simply a collection of neural circuits in the brain that have gone awry, that have been hijacked by addiction. It weaves such a remarkable illusion of selfhood that we refer to it as a "self," or the "false self." But this is just a rhetorical convenience – because there is no self at the center of the addiction persona. If the addiction persona were a "self," its identity and purpose would be purely one-dimensional: it sends you into survival mode when your survival is not significantly at risk. And that's *all* it does. Its complexity comes from the various ways it can hijack and manipulate different parts of you to serve that basic purpose. But despite its almost unfathomable destructiveness, it doesn't pursue this end intentionally or maliciously. The effect just *happens*. It's an emergent property of the brain, a trick, an illusion.

The addiction persona can seem like an evil demon that's always concocting a plan to draw you back into addiction. But that's only because survival-mode states create such a powerful magnetic pull, both from the primal, existential fear of death that the states trigger, and from the substantial biochemical payoffs that they supply. Believe it or not, the addiction persona is actually trying to *help* you. Things just get mixed up. The addiction persona is like a deer that has walked through an open door in a modern suburban store and is wandering through the aisles, desperate, frightened, and lost in the way many people are lost. The deer could just walk over to the door and gently push it open to be free again, but it doesn't know where the door is or how to open it. So it jumps through the storefront window and badly injures itself. That's what addiction and the addiction persona are like.

The addiction persona also consistently seeks to justify the states of survival mode that it continually throws us into. The tendency for us to justify our behavior, even if that behavior is frankly unethical or destructive, appears to be part of the brain's original design. The addiction persona, however, corrupts and hijacks this normal function to a highly unnatural degree. Part of the brain is also clearly designed to create narratives that offer at least somewhat reasonable explanations for circumstances that we find ourselves in, or for decisions we find ourselves making. The addiction persona corrupts and misuses this capacity as well.

The psychiatrist Albert Moll used hypnosis to show how people can readily create justifications for even the most bizarre behavior. In one of his experiments, Moll suggested to a man under hypnosis that when the man emerged from his hypnotic state, he was to "take a flower-pot from the window, wrap it in a cloth, put it on the sofa, and bow to it three times." The subject dutifully performed this sequence directly after being released from his hypnotic state. When the man was asked why he had carried out these completely arbitrary actions he said, as Moll reported: "You know, when I woke and saw the flower-pot there I thought that as it was rather cold the flower-pot had better be warmed a little, or else the plant would die. So I wrapped it in the cloth, and then I thought that as the sofa was near the fire I would put the flowerpot on it; and I bowed because I was pleased with myself for having such a bright idea."

The addiction persona similarly creates far-fetched justifications for even the most destructive addiction-driven behavior: the compulsive drinking of the alcoholic who is ruining his career and his relationships, or the compulsive worrying of a woman who spends most of her days being anxious rather than living her life. All of us apparently *need* to have a story to make sense of our lives and the circumstances we find ourselves in. When we're functional, this story is the very best we can discern about the world and our role in it, the story closest to the truth as far as we can tell. We don't lie to ourselves by telling a false story – our story about ourselves and our situation is simply the best, truest, and most functional story that we're capable of telling at that time. As we'll discuss more in Chapter 9, the addiction persona creates stories that, although often clever, are clearly false – not only to the more observant people around us, but even to part of ourselves.

The addiction persona sends us unnecessarily into distressing, out-of-balance states just to get a paltry and corrupted payoff. Since this is a fundamentally irrational pursuit, it requires deceit, lies, and false justifications in order to be carried out. Therefore anything related to addiction is always founded in illusion, in falseness. Addiction is a remarkably powerful driving force when we are unconscious of how it operates, but as soon as we become conscious of its inner workings, of its essential nature, it becomes increasingly weaker. To truly overcome its effects, however, we have to find all of its hiding places, we have to shine the light of our consciousness on all the nooks and crannies of the psyche to see where addiction might be hiding.

As we've seen, addiction in its simplest form takes negative emotions like anxiety or worry and then uses and exaggerates those emotions just to get a drug payoff. But it can also take *positive* emotions and use and exaggerate *them* by creating false states of survival mode. Perhaps most of all, the addiction persona corrupts *feeling*, emotions, aliveness. It takes anything that is potentially blissful, anything that is potentially authentic and homeostatic, and saps the bliss, the life from it by making it inauthentic, forced, and illusory. Anything – even love – can be corrupted by addiction.

Addiction may unconsciously trick you, for example, into believing that if you lose someone you love, you literally will die – that you *need* that other person in order to survive. Addiction can also manipulate love in more subtle ways. Many people, for instance, are naturally very caring and loving. But what addiction might do is unconsciously convince some of these people that they need to be even *more* loving than what comes naturally to them for them to be "enough," for them not to be or feel "less than." These people may then become "caretakers" in their relationships, in that they exaggerate their natural attribute of being caring because they believe, at least at some level, that they wouldn't be able to maintain those relationships without their unnatural investment in the role of being a caretaker. In other words, addiction, in this case, effectively makes being loving and caring about *survival*. If you're not exceptionally loving, addiction warns you, you may lose your important relationships – or, in a more primal, unconscious sense, you might get thrown out of the band, or might not be able to successfully mate.

If you lose important relationships as a hunter-gatherer, you really might die. If you lose important relationships in modern life, it's always extremely painful – but very rarely are you going to die just from those losses. This is how addiction distorts us: it makes all of our experiences and emotions, even love, about survival. Addiction is always trying to shift us into survival mode.

The addiction persona is also fed by unsettling, disconnecting thoughts. It is impossible for us to be balanced, for example, if we are constantly worried about what other people think of us. We have no *control* over what other people may or may not be thinking. And so if our self-worth, our sense of feeling okay, is dependent on the judgments of other people, we will *always* be out of balance, because our sense of balance, our homeostasis, will always be at the mercy of forces we have no control over. Most of us also often create "false projections" in which we attribute thoughts or intentions to other people that clearly don't reflect that person's true thoughts or intentions. False projections can create powerful illusions. We might feel absolutely certain that another person has a certain thought or point of view and be completely wrong.

False projections almost always operate in the service of addiction. That is, when we unconsciously project inaccurate feelings, beliefs, or judgments onto other people, particularly when the projections create distress in us, we are acting out of the addictive drive. False projections driven by the addiction persona seem to be largely responsible for the veil of illusion that frequently clouds most people's vision – what Buddhists call "Maya."

To overcome all the pernicious effects of the addiction persona, we need to be fully aware of the many ways it can trigger us into different states of survival mode. Our greatest tool in dissolving the addiction persona, in overcoming and transcending its effects, is consciousness. This book and the model it describes are intended to increase your consciousness, to give you the tools you need to dissolve the addiction persona. The first step is to understand the theory – to see the distinction between a healthy biochemical reward and an unhealthy drug payoff, between authentic emotions and emotions that are being exaggerated or manufactured just to derive an artificial drug payoff.

Translating this theory into practice, into informing the decisions you actually make in your life, is admittedly more challenging. It takes practice. But if you can always hold the theory in your mind, you will be guided towards a solution to your own unique situation. The homeostatic drive and the True Self will guide you; every piece of this model and system that you can absorb – the theory as well as other tools we'll present – will further dissolve the false self while strengthening the True Self and the homeostatic drive.

One of the clearest manifestations of the homeostatic drive is a state of "flow." A pure state of flow can come from almost any activity, almost any circumstance. But it is most frequently experienced during acts of creation, such as writing or painting, or during feelings of emotional connection with another person, or during any type of play or satisfying work. The most critical aspect of a state of flow is complete absorption in what you're doing. When you're in flow, the present moment cascades before you and within you – the present moment does indeed feel eternal. When you're in flow, you don't care what other people may or may not be thinking about you; you're absorbed in your own experience, your own aliveness.

Pure states of flow are extremely weakening to the addiction persona. States of flow typically send a clear message to the brain that our survival is *not at risk*. And if the state of flow involves an inherently dangerous activity – such as rock-climbing – this particular state will send a message to the brain that you are confronting *real* risks to your survival, not illusory ones. States of flow relax the addiction persona. The addiction persona, in a sense, itself becomes caught up in the intoxicating state of flow, and is soothed and distracted, like Frankenstein being calmed by the sound of beautiful, distant music.

But because the addiction persona feeds on the force that opposes states of flow, it will, in effect – and only in effect – tend to fight against flow states and the drive that gives rise to those flow states. The addiction persona will act to reinforce its *own* neural circuits – the circuits that create disconnection, pain, judgment, obsession with the future and the past. However, it doesn't fear so much for its *own* survival – it fears for *yours*. It keeps throwing you into survival mode out of a misguided desire to protect *you*. That's the irony. Although its over-protectiveness frequently manifests as abusiveness, or even as evil itself, the addiction persona isn't at all malicious. It simply becomes swept up in the illusion that it itself is largely responsible for creating.

Although we've been discussing the addiction persona up to this point as if it were one entity, it can actually be further subdivided. Just as people with multiple personality disorder (now often called dissociative identity disorder) have different "alters," or alternate personalities, the addiction persona is also composed of alternative false selves. Whenever you exhibit an addictive behavior, that behavior will be performed, in effect, by an alter that is specific for that particular addiction.

If something painful happens to you – someone important to you rejects you, for example, or ignores you, doesn't respond to you the way you might like – you might start to feel "less than." This feeling can act as a trigger that sends you into an addiction alter. Different people will respond in different ways to "less than" triggers. Some may activate a sex addiction alter. Others may overeat. Others may become overtly self-pitying, recalling many other times in their lives that they felt unbearably "less than." While they're obsessively revisiting these painful memories, their bodies might be slumped, their shoulders raised, their jaws clenched. Each of these dysfunctional behavioral patterns is driven by a distinct addiction alter that becomes reinforced by the drug payoffs that the alter delivers. The alter is disconnected from the authentic self. It is associated with specific memories, a specific type of false self-image, a specific type of body posture, a specific kind of compulsion. It is very much like an alternative personality. The alters have a dysfunctional, distorted view of your self and of the world that feed into the addiction that they facilitate, and so they tell you a distorted story about the circumstances surrounding the triggering of your pain.

In a hunter-gatherer context, the feeling of self-pity, for example, would probably only be activated by a physical or emotional injury that truly threatened survival. If you felt and expressed self-pity in this context, it would probably be, at least in large part, a desperate attempt to draw the attention of other people towards your plight, a desperate plea for their support. Self-pity is simply another manifestation of being in survival mode.

Alters are usually generated in early childhood, when the perception, and perhaps in some cases the reality, was that they really did help you to survive. Perhaps being self-pitying, for example, was the only thing that got you the attention from your parents that you craved. For children, attention is perceived as a critical survival need. Part of the brain, therefore, thinks that self-pity once saved your life; and so, unconsciously, you often revert back to that state when you're triggered into survival mode. All animals, including humans, revert to old ingrained patterns when survival is at risk, because, in the wild, these old patterns often provide the best chance for survival. But with addiction, old painful patterns are re-engaged *dysfunctionally*, when survival is *not* at risk. Hence addiction-driven patterns only serve to perpetuate unnecessary states of pain, distress, and survival mode. Rather than helping us to survive, to live, addiction alters *keep* us from living.

Addiction alters are driven by neural networks in the brain that have become dysfunctional. When those neural networks are activated, they draw you further into your pain by telling lies to you about yourself, by manipulating your self-image, distorting your view of yourself. They distort your past by preferentially activating all of your most painful memories, and very frequently distort the memories themselves. If distorted memories don't make you feel sufficiently "less than" – or self-pitying or angry – the alter may drive you into fantasies, or "anti-fantasies," of painful, imaginary situations, or it may lead you to project thoughts onto other people that make you feel exceptionally awful. You may imagine that certain people, for example, are almost constantly laughing at you behind your back, looking down at you, disrespecting you.

Alters often arise from childhood traumas such as physical, sexual, or emotional abuse. But they can also arise from more subtle childhood traumas, such as receiving too little care or attention, or from adult traumas such as a war trauma, rape, a painful breakup, or some perceived betrayal. Every trauma that happens to us needs to be processed, accepted, and somehow integrated with the rest of us. We don't need to be defined by that trauma, but we need to accept that it happened to us, we need to accept that it is part of our history. If a trauma isn't integrated in this way, it will become split off, discon-nected – it will become an alter. If we've processed and accepted the trauma, we can think of it months or years later without undue pain – with acceptance, or perhaps even with gratitude for how it led to our growth as human beings. But if the trauma is not processed and accepted, when we later think about it or are reminded of it by specific circumstances, we'll often be triggered into an alter that's specific for that trauma. The trauma will have a magnetic pull that keeps drawing us back to it. That pull comes from the huge biochemical payoffs that reengaging in the trauma will supply, and is sustained because any trauma by its nature is a circumstance that sent us into survival mode. So when the trauma is re-activated, we'll feel like we're once again experiencing some sort of survival threat. That's the illusion – very rarely is it the reality.

In the most severe cases, alters become so disconnected that they result in multiple personality disorder (MPD). With MPD, a person's alters are so disconnected from primary consciousness that the person may develop amnesia for anything the alter does. The alter almost literally begins to live separately from the actual person. The most famous case of MPD became the subject of the book and movie "Sybil," and the phenomenon has since been repeatedly confirmed by a number of other clinical studies with other patients.

Nearly all of us, however, have the same dynamic operating within us, although typically to a far less severe degree. The tricky thing about addiction alters is that they almost always involve something that really *is* part of you. If you experienced a trauma in the past, that trauma is part of you, part of your history, your experience. Similarly, sex addiction or food addiction alters contain authentic elements of the self. Embedded in a person's sex addiction alter is a healthy sexuality; part of the neural network that drives a person's food addiction alter would, if expressed in another context, drive a healthy desire for food, and an authentic and healthy appreciation for the pleasure and sense of well-being that food can bring. Beneath every "caretaker" addiction is an authentically caring human being. Within each addiction alter, a split-off portion of the True Self is hidden like a diamond.

Although few of us have a condition as severe as Sybil's, nearly all of us have our own version of it. Nearly all of us have at least several dysfunctional alters. As we'll discuss more in Chapter 10, the first step in breaking down your addiction alters is to identify the specific type of addictive patterns they are responsible for. The second step is to identify the *triggers* that commonly trigger you into the addictive patterns. The third step is to create a panel, or set, of what we call "neural antibodies" (discussed further in Chapter 11). Just as

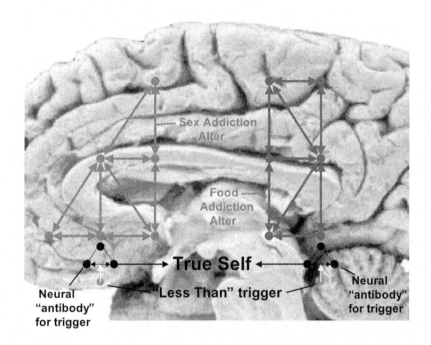

Figure 6: A schematic representation of "neural antibodies" and neural networks that drive food and sex addiction "alters." "Neural antibodies" are thought patterns that intercept triggers which might otherwise trigger addictive patterns, or "alters." Neural antibodies will effectively re-route the trigger back to neural networks that support homeostatic patterns and the True Self.

an antibody in the immune system recognizes a foreign pathogen like a bacterium or a virus, and then kills the pathogen and expels it from the body, a "neural" antibody is a thought pattern that "attaches to" the trigger to keep it from activating the addiction alter (Figure 6). Since the addiction persona as a whole relies on illusions and false-hoods for its existence, a neural antibody is a thought pattern that reinforces the *truth* about you and your circumstances. Ideally, a neural antibody involves a deep emotion you've experienced that reinforces an *emotional* truth about yourself – the neural antibody could, for example, reinforce the profound pain you experienced or caused to others as a result of your addiction, whether that addiction involves alcohol, drugs, sex, food, or any other destructive emotional or behavioral pattern.

If you can create and consistently mobilize these neural antibodies – if you can have them, in effect, in your "circulation" – you can keep the addiction alters from becoming activated. The general rule in the brain is "use it or lose it." If you continually activate an addiction alter, or any other neural network, it will become stronger – it will become easier and easier to activate, and will become more and more reinforced in the brain. But if you can use your panel of neural antibodies to keep the alters from being triggered, the alters will grow weaker. If you can successfully live for extended periods without triggering the alters, it's quite possible that the neural networks that drive the alters may disappear entirely. In dissolving an alter, you will be at the same time recovering the elements of the True Self that were embedded in the alter, and you can then connect this new healthy neural network to the rest of you. Because the addiction persona is composed of various addiction alters, this process will slowly dissolve the addiction persona, and slowly reinforce and uncover the True Self. And the ultimate goal of the healing system described in this book is nothing less than the full uncovering and realization of the True Self.

The True Self is typically split apart in early childhood, dispersed in sections that become overseen by various addiction alters, and by the addiction persona as a whole. For most of us, that overseeing voice of the addiction persona is almost always looming, almost always speaking softly in the background. When you're weak, when you're stressed, or hurt, or out of balance, the addiction persona's voice becomes louder and more insistent, trying to drag you further into your pain, trying to coax you even further out of balance. It's when you're disconnected from the True Self that the old traumas come back and start to really pull at you, drawing you back into survival mode, into the maelstrom, into that old hurt.

Being in survival mode is usually to feel like a victim. When we become caught in an addictive loop, we typically feel like victims because forces beyond our awareness or apparent control appear to keep sending us, or forcing us, into survival mode. But those forces come from *us*, or from the "false," or addiction persona, part of us. The addiction persona always feels like a victim also, however, because it is always acting out of a survival emergency, out of forces that it is confused by, that it consistently misinterprets.

Although the addiction persona causes you so much pain, it doesn't intend you any harm. It's just a misunderstanding, a mistake, a glitch in the operating system that needs to be repaired and rewired. Everything the addiction persona does it does because it's looking out for your survival. It just gets confused; it thinks that your survival is threatened when, in actuality, you're relatively safe. The addiction persona is like a Neanderthal who's been assigned to look after you and is trying to adapt to the bustling, modern commercial culture in which you live. It's trained to hunt wildebeests with a spear and now you want it to sit down in a busy restaurant and eat sushi with chopsticks. It becomes afraid and befuddled, and it always screams the same thing: we're all going to die. The addiction persona is stuck in one gear, and that gear is always survival mode.

CHAPTER 8

RELATIONSHIP DRAMAS

Dysfunctional relationship "dramas" are an extremely important and widespread manifestation of emotional addiction. When we're operating out of emotional addiction within ourselves, we cause ourselves pain and throw ourselves out of balance with our own thoughts and behavior. In a relationship drama, one or both partners frequently seek, consciously or unconsciously, to throw *each other* out of balance or cause *each other* pain or distress. Any emotional or physical drama involves heightened emotional states that release substantial amounts of dopamine and endorphin into reward areas. Relationship dramas can therefore become a powerful way of delivering huge drug payoffs to the brain.

Just as any of us can derive biochemical payoffs from our own pain and emotional "drama," we can also clearly derive payoffs from other people's pain under some circumstances. We can cause other people emotional pain either actively – by insulting them or making them feel "less than," for example; or passively – by trying, for example, to make them feel guilty. We human beings can do with language and emotional manipulation what other animals do physically – we bite, scratch, hurt, and pummel each other.

In general, however, other people's pain will only be satisfying to us if part of us feels that those people, at least at some level, *deserve* their pain and suffering. If they did or said something to hurt or harm us or someone we care about, for example, that may trigger us into seeking revenge in some form. Brain imaging experiments have shown how this general dynamic appears to work. Studies involving games where money is exchanged between two players according to specified rules and agreements, have shown that observers of the games express emotional satisfaction, and even pleasure, when players who act unfairly or unethically receive electric shocks. As the observers either watch the electric shocks being delivered to the unethical player, or as they themselves administer the electric shocks, reward areas in their brains become strongly activated, especially in those observers who express a distinct desire for revenge against the unethical player.

People in intimate relationships will almost unavoidably hurt each other emotionally on occasion. And it's easy for us to feel that the hurt we've suffered at the hands of a person close to us was somehow intentional, conscious, or even unethical – even though it may seem quite obvious to outside observers that the cause of the injury was accidental, incidental, or unconscious. This is a common illusion: we feel intense pain in response to something another person says or does and we directly associate our pain with the person's conscious *intention* to cause us pain.

Of course, sometimes people *do* have this conscious intention, but far more often they do not. The great likelihood is that when we're hurt by other people, those people were themselves acting unconsciously out of some state of survival mode. Or they were simply making a choice or decision that, for their own reasons and given their own situations, they honestly felt compelled to make. Because of this common association between our pain and another person's apparently malicious intent, which various projections can allow to seem so *real*, we can easily justify hurting people we care deeply about after we ourselves have been hurt.

Almost anyone can potentially throw us out of balance. But the people closest to us – especially our family members, spouses, or lovers – can really *blast* us out of balance. Partly this is because our relationships with them are so important to us, and partly it's because they know where we are most vulnerable. They always know, for example, how they can trigger us into a nice, turbulent drama. The healthiest relationships have little or no unnecessary drama, however, and the relationship almost always helps both people find their way back to homeostasis when they become distressed.

Losing important relationships can trigger some of the worst pain that human beings can suffer. And just as it's critical for our emotional health to seek human connection, it's completely appropriate to be pained or distraught when important connections are lost. What we don't want to do, however, is to *linger* in that pain any longer than we need to; we don't want to *use* that pain to get a drug payoff. We also don't want to fall under the illusion that our survival will be at risk because of the loss, because this will very rarely be the case, particularly once we become adults. The loss of someone we're attached to may be extremely painful, and it may take time for us to come back into homeostasis after such a loss. But only very rarely is that loss going to be a significant survival risk for us.

The intense pain we can feel from the loss of important relationships is largely due to our hunter-gatherer heritage. Hunter-gatherers have no bank accounts or secure homes, no emergency supplies of canned or frozen food. They only have each other: they rely on their *relationships* for their survival. This is why we're biologically wired to invest so much in our close relationships, and why we can feel so distraught and bereft when those relationships end or are damaged. During our long evolutionary history as hunter-gatherers, close relationships were absolutely essential for our survival, and that evolutionary history is still encoded in our genes, our psyches, and in our general sense of emotional stability.

Our evolutionary history has also left a strong tendency in us to perpetuate relationship patterns we were exposed to as infants and children. Since nearly all behavioral patterns in hunter-gatherers are functional, when hunter-gatherers repeat the relationship patterns they were exposed to as children, those repeated patterns are also likely to be functional. But in the modern world, many of our childhood experiences occur in the midst of extreme dysfunction, and so if the relationship patterns arising from *those* experiences are repeated, the original dysfunctions will only be perpetuated and even compounded.

Women who suffer through chronic abuse, for example, have almost always been seriously abused as children. While there's never any excuse or acceptable justification for abuse of any kind, the reality is that most women who are repeatedly abused by their boyfriends or husbands typically bear about half of the responsibility for the abuse. Abusers are one hundred percent wrong for their reprehensible acts, and they are one hundred percent accountable for those acts. But women who are consistently and repeatedly abused are almost always attracted at some level to abusive men, and almost always repeatedly place themselves in situations that can easily lead to their being abused. This is a consequence of unconscious addictive dynamics that are no "fault" of the woman, or really of anyone else. Nearly all women who allow themselves to be abused as adults were severely abused as children and thus were at grave risk for developing a biochemical addiction to the trauma of abuse. So while the healthy part of them – the True Self – will want to find nurturing relationships, the unhealthy, addictive part of them – the addiction persona, or addiction alters – will unconsciously seek out abuse so that the addiction dynamic can be perpetuated. The same is true for men who dysfunctionally seek emotionally abusive women.

Chronically abused women receive enormous drug payoffs from the cycle of abuse: from the intense fear they feel when the abuser becomes enraged; from the intense feelings of self-pity, victimhood, and rage they experience during the abuse; and from the temporary, although delusional, sense of safety they feel during each reconciliation. When we are children and are utterly dependent on our parents or caregivers for our survival, there are only a limited number of choices we can make that will influence our circumstances. But when we're adults, an enormous range of options typically stand before us, particularly about the kinds of people we choose to associate with. Victimhood, at least in adults who live in modern democratic societies, is almost always an illusion. Random hurtful or damaging events can happen to anyone, but repeated abuse almost always requires our complicity. Under most circumstances, if we are consistently abused as adults, at some level we must be conspiring in that abuse – we must be *allowing* ourselves to be abused out of addiction.

This is not at all to "blame the victim." We're not blaming *anyone*. These are all dynamics that just *happen*, either wholly or largely unconsciously. People who fall into addictive patterns that are destructive to themselves and to others are almost always people who are not conscious of how these dynamics operate. Very few people, if they truly understood the dynamics that drive them to act destructively, would consciously and knowingly choose to hurt themselves or other people unnecessarily. Abusive people must be held accountable for what they do, just as people who commit murder must go to prison. But it makes no more sense to "blame" or "judge" what an unconscious person does than it does to blame someone for what they do while they're sleepwalking. Destructive people are almost always caught in addiction-driven forces that they don't understand and that they become profoundly tricked by.

One useful system for analyzing dysfunctional relationship interactions views the interactions as "control dramas." The interactions are called "control" dramas because when people engage in such dramas, they are, in effect, unconsciously trying to manipulate, or "control" another person into assuming a complementary drama, or role, so that they themselves can get a dysfunctional biochemical payoff from the dynamic.

Each of the four control drama roles – "intimidator," "interrogator," "aloof," and "poor me" – can be seen as a type of false self, or addiction alter. Interrogators ask a lot of probing questions, and always feel better when they can find fault with, and hence feel "more than," other people. In romantic relationships in particular, interrogators will very often attract aloofs, and aloofs will attract interrogators. The aloof type doesn't readily offer love or affection, and tends to withdraw physically and emotionally, generally interacting with people in an oblique way. Their aloofness is very distressing to interrogators.

An intimidator gets a dysfunctional payoff from bullying or hurting a "poor me." And a "poor me" gets a dysfunctional payoff from self-pity, and from making an intimidator feel guilty, or like a "bad" person. The intimidator and "poor me" dramas are therefore complementary, or opposite, types. The interrogator and aloof types are also complementary. In the great majority of cases, the romantic relationships people voluntarily choose to have, particularly if they are unaware of how control drama dynamics operate, will be with their opposite type.

Each person's role in a control drama encourages and enables the expression of the complementary role. Although interrogators, for example, don't like it when aloofs are distracted or disengaged, interrogators can behave in ways that tend to trigger even more aloofness in their already aloof partners. Aloofs get their dysfunctional payoffs by, for example, driving an interrogator to follow them around the house yelling: "Listen to me! Don't walk away from me! We need to talk about this!" This kind of outburst from an interrogator will generally cause the aloof to be even more disengaged, which will in turn make the interrogator even more furious, and thus perpetuate the whole drama. Interrogators and aloofs often drive each other crazy, but they can be very attracted to each other because they both get enormous biochemical payoffs from their dynamic, and those payoffs will potentiate any sexual attraction they may already have for each other. Because the participants in the drama consistently send each other into survival mode, the illusion is also created that there's some sort of overriding urgency to the relationship – that their lives may literally depend on it.

Control drama styles are almost always derived from our relationship with our parents or primary caregivers, although sometimes also from our relationships with siblings or other relatives. These influences start at the earliest stages of infancy, and continue through childhood. Typically, a child will either model or oppose the control dramas of the dominant parent, the parent who has the most emotional impact on the child. But although a father, for example, may hardly ever be home, his extreme *absence* may be what makes him the dominant influence on the development of the control dramas of his children, because his absence is likely to be profoundly traumatic and unsettling. If the father's primary control drama, for example, is intimidator and his secondary control drama is aloof, some of his children may model him by assuming the same control dramas as him. Other children may oppose him by having "poor me" as their primary control drama, and interrogator as their secondary control drama. In the great majority of cases, this seems to be how the dynamic works, with occasional exceptions and variations on the general theme.

In a real sense, a child has no say in what control drama he or she develops. It all happens unconsciously, and it begins to happen while the child is an infant. There's probably a significant genetic component to whether a child will model or oppose the dominant parent. Children who are genetically predisposed to being very fearful or timid, for example, are probably more prone to being "poor me," while children who are genetically predisposed to being more aggressive and fearless are more likely to become intimidators.

It's important to realize, however, that, although nearly everyone has one or two control dramas that are especially prominent, nearly all of us can potentially express all four of the control dramas, all four of the addiction "alters," at different times. We've all been conditioned to keep using the control dramas that have been giving us the most payoffs and that, when we were children, created the unconscious impression that they enhanced our survival prospects. In modern, Western culture, in particular, parental dynamics with children almost always contain a substantial amount of dysfunction. And since any dysfunction, almost by definition, will be interpreted by an infant or young child as a true survival threat, control drama dynamics become interwoven with primal fears during childhood, particularly the fear of abandonment.

All the dramas are in their own specific ways difficult to deal with. The "poor me" dynamic, for example, can challenge our compassion. When you detect someone "using" their feelings of self-pity to manipulate some response from you, or to simply to get a drug payoff within themselves, it's very easy to forget that, for them, those painful feelings are quite real, although their pain is being unconsciously exaggerated to enhance the drug payoff. When we're confronted with a "poor me," there's often part of us that can be triggered into sadistically wanting to beat up or pick on the "poor me," like a cruel child picking on a more vulnerable child.

In a hunter-gatherer context, engaging in any of the four control dramas would be an indicator of desperately low status – that is, of feeling "less than," and interpreting that feeling as representing a true survival threat. Like all addictions, control dramas are dysfunctional imitations of behavior patterns that in a natural context would be functional. If a hunter-gatherer man is injured emotionally or physically, for example, his feeling of "poor me" could well lead to his receiving more food or attention from other band members who feel sorry for him. "Poor me" is a submissive posture – it's like an animal rolling on its back to expose its vulnerable belly to you, an act of submission, that asks for your sympathy, forbearance, and mercy. Feelings and expressions of "poor me" in various circumstances probably saved the lives of hundreds of thousands of hunter-gatherers in our evolutionary past, and so the unconscious pattern became incorporated into the behavioral tendencies that are our biological birthright.

A hunter-gatherer who has a comfortable and stable level of status in the group, however, would probably rarely, if ever, resort to *any* of the control dramas. People who are truly confident don't need to prove themselves by intimidating or interrogating other people to try to make themselves feel "more than." If these people sometimes seem aloof, that aloofness is *authentic*, it arises from something they truly feel. They're not being aloof so that they'll get a dysfunctional payoff from tormenting an interrogator. They just are who they are, and are not trying to present a false image of themselves to manipulate a response from other people. Needing to present such an image is a desperate, "less than," low-status tactic, like a low-status monkey smiling ingratiatingly to avoid getting beaten up by a dominant monkey. A low-status monkey needs to watch what it does, and needs to be careful about how dominant animals respond to its behavior. When we feel "less than," we tap into those same primal fears. The key difference between hunter-gatherers and people who live in modern, industrialized cultures, however, is that the survival of people in the modern world is far less at risk from their status level. That's the disconnect.

Relationships are always infinitely more fulfilling if we don't approach them as a compensation for addiction-driven feelings of "less than." Ideally, any relationship is simply an opportunity to connect with another human being. Control dramas, on the other hand, are not about true connection – they're about getting drug payoffs from states that are driven by an unconscious survival response. When you're in a full-fledged, knock-down control drama with another person, it's very much like two false selves, two addiction alters, having a senseless battle. The drama is inauthentic, absurd, and highly destructive. Control dramas often become about being *right*, about *winning*. You want to show the other person they're wrong and you want to show them *why* they're wrong. Arguments within a control drama usually just become about throwing the other person out of balance or hurting them.

The key to overcoming control dramas is accepting that you only have power over your *own* role in the drama. By focusing on your own part in the drama, you'll withdraw most of the fuel that has been keeping the drama crackling and burning. The other person who has been a co-conspirator in the drama will then see that you're no longer doing what you have typically done, and will be motivated to relax his or her own role in the drama.

In any control drama, it's very easy to place responsibility on the *other* person in the drama, to focus on them. But the only thing that liberates us from control dramas is to focus on *ourselves*, on our own complicity in the drama, and to admit that we ourselves are allowing the drama to be perpetuated. If we weren't getting a biochemical payoff from the drama, we wouldn't allow ourselves to keep getting drawn back into it.

When you begin to take ownership of your own role in a control drama, it often has to be an almost aggressive protection of yourself – that you will *not* allow the other person to make you feel "less than," angry, or anxious. If you do feel any of these negative emotions, you'll know that their unconscious control tactics worked! And if their tactics worked, that tells you that you still have work to do. You have to take ownership and, in effect, say to the other person: you can't make me feel "less than," or angry; your unconscious behavior cannot make me become unconscious.

This becomes far more challenging when a person close to you is trying to engage you in a control drama that you're particularly susceptible to. They're threatening to send you into survival mode, and offering you a drug that part of you still craves, but that you've also tagged as a drug that is profoundly unhealthy for you. These are supposed to be people who care about you and they're almost forcing you, seemingly at knife-point, to go into a painful emergency state and take this unhealthy drug! So it's easy to get angry with them. What is more difficult, at least at first, but ultimately far more healthy, is to see that you can only take responsibility for your *own* part in the control drama. You have no control over *them*, and, if you're healthy, you don't want control over them. You need to become clear that what other people do is about *them*, it's a reflection of *them*, and it's not a reflection of you or your own worth.

Your job is to grow and evolve so that you eventually find a way not to be triggered into your control dramas under any circumstance. And this takes a great deal of consciousness – consciousness about how your control dramas operate, what triggers you into them, and consciousness about how the things *you* do may trigger an impulse in other people that can motivate them to try to sweep you into their own control dramas. It isn't easy, but it does become easier and easier the more you work at it, and the more you see that you can only be responsible for your own part in the drama. When you really begin to understand that you have fifty percent of the responsibility for any control drama you engage in, you're well on your way to overcoming your particular control drama addictions.

Control drama relationship dynamics with family members and significant others have addictive elements that are every bit as strong as addiction to cigarettes or cocaine. And in some ways, control dramas can be even harder to deal with than addiction to drugs, partly because the dynamics become ingrained during early childhood, a period we typically have little or no memory of. But remember that if you can become the master of yourself in any control dynamic, the dynamic will automatically begin to shift. It's extremely unlikely that the other person in the dynamic will be instantly "healed," or that they will do exactly what you want them to do. But the dynamic will be different, and it will be healthier.

When you're in a control drama, you're getting a drug payoff not only by hurting yourself, but also by hurting someone else. You're unconsciously manipulating another person into an emotional state that is often very painful to them. Once you become fully conscious of how control dramas work, it's difficult to keep engaging in them, because you see how irresponsible they are, and how injurious the dynamic can be – particularly to people who are especially vulnerable emotionally and physically. You can't blame yourself for how you acted before you were conscious of control drama dynamics. You just didn't *know*. You did the best you could with what you thought to be true, with what you were conscious of, what you understood and believed at that time. But once you know, you have to take responsibility for that knowledge.

A person in a control drama with you may well have the unconscious or half-conscious intent of manipulating you, of wanting to have power over you. But if you have a strong physiological reaction to their attempt, that only shows you that you are still deeply immersed in the drama yourself. *You* have to take responsibility for that physiological reaction and take action or make decisions or increase consciousness within yourself so that you can heal your addiction to that particular pattern. Because whenever you have such a strong physiological reaction, your stress response will be triggered, and whenever your stress response is triggered, you receive a drug. So, in this circumstance, you still have to accept the reality that part of you, either unconsciously or half-consciously, is using this control drama opportunity to allow yourself to be thrown unnecessarily into survival mode and to receive a drug. Furthermore, when the other person in the drama with you *sees* that you have a physiological reaction to the drama, *they* will get a charge, a payoff, from that as well, and the addictive loop of the control drama will only be reinforced – not only for you, but for them as well.

When you start to become conscious of control drama dynamics, you may well feel it as a turning point in your own emotional and spiritual development. But then another trap typically awaits you. It becomes very easy to be excessively angry with and unsympathetic towards the people who are unconsciously trying to draw you back into a control drama. The more conscious you become, and the easier it becomes for you to perceive control drama dynamics, the easier it will be for you to think that other people should just *get* it. Once you see and understand the dynamic, it all seems so obvious. Something else to keep in mind is that while control dramas, like all addictions, can be very easy to see in *other* people, they're typically far more difficult to see in ourselves. Unless we're being constantly videotaped as we make our way in the world, we'll never be able see ourselves or our own facial expressions or body postures the way other people can as they observe us. Since we can't observe ourselves from the outside, we can potentially develop a severely skewed perspective on ourselves and on our own behavior.

Another potential trap you may fall into after confronting your control dramas is that it's easy at first to swing in the opposite direction and try to avoid *all* conflict with other people. While unnecessary conflict is always undesirable, and always arises from addiction, sometimes conflicts are authentic and need to be resolved in the healthiest way possible. That is, two people in any relationship may have conflicting goals or beliefs, and somehow those differences need to be acknowledged, resolved, and brought into homeostasis. If the conflicts can't be reconciled, that should be admitted by both parties, and in some cases the only homeostatic solution is to end or fundamentally change the nature of the relationship.

If you want the other person in the relationship, for their own benefit and for yours, to change the way they operate, it will also almost always be counter-productive to make it your passion and purpose to have them change. This in itself is likely to set up *another* drama in which you're trying to change them – in effect to *control* them – and they're trying to resist you. Having this kind of conscious or unconscious *agenda* with someone you're in a relationship with will almost always create some sort of drama between the two of you. If you have an agenda, even if it isn't frankly stated, it will always show up in your emotional and physical posture, in your overall energy.

When someone has an agenda towards you, you always feel that tug from them, that impulse to shape and control you, which the healthy part of you will resist. People who have an agenda towards you, who want or need you to respond to them in a specific way, can never just be vulnerable and authentic with you. When we have an agenda of trying to "fix" someone without their consent, and our agenda sets up a control drama dynamic with them, the very thing we want will often be exactly what they are going to resist.

But if you show up in the relationship with no judgment and with no agenda except to stay focused on your *own* control dramas, and just to be authentic and connected to yourself in every moment, the power of the control drama will begin to weaken. The other person will likely continue to bait you, throw their usual barbs at you, but if you're fully conscious, and are assuming full responsibility for your own role in the dynamic, then the other person in the dynamic will ultimately lose the drive to operate in the way he or she did previously. Control dramas are almost always very challenging, partly because they're such powerful addictions, and partly because they involve other people whom we have no control over, but whom we are often deeply attached to.

Ideally we would all be in relationships with people we truly care about and connect to, with people we truly love and feel loved by, people who meet some of our authentic, core needs. As we begin to heal the addictive patterns that both arise from and perpetuate feelings of "less than," we become far less prone to getting into relationships with other people just because, for example, those people are perceived to have high status. *Needing* to have a relationship with someone who has high status is just another "less than" compensation – a dysfunctional way for a person who feels "less than" to try to feel "more than." The healthiest payoffs in relationships come simply from connecting with another person, from giving and receiving love in a way that nourishes the expression and realization of the True Self in both of you. Everything else is just a drama.

CHAPTER 9

BELIEF SYSTEMS AND PERSONAL "STORIES"

Just as people who live in their natural state as hunter-gatherers are rarely neurotic, psychotic, or otherwise dysfunctional, animals too are almost always functional in the wild. But when animals are forced to live in highly unnatural conditions – particularly when they're put in cages for extended periods – they often begin to behave in ways that have all the hallmarks of addiction to pain and distress. Chimpanzees who are put in a cage alone will often bite their own leg until the leg bleeds, or pull out their own hair, or bang their heads against the bars of the cage. Just as modern industrialized environments are radically unnatural for people, being in a cage alone is completely unnatural for any animal. Since living in a cage is something animals would never encounter in the wild, it is an experience that evolution has not prepared them for, and the experience can often trigger addictive patterns.

We modern humans tend to live in cages also, but the cages are usually constructed from our *belief systems*, our dysfunctional "stories" about ourselves. How do you know if your belief system is dysfunctional? When it causes you unnecessary pain and distress, when it throws you unnecessarily into various types of survival mode, and when it simply isn't *true*. Dysfunctional belief systems, upon close analysis, are never rational, they never really make any sense. Addiction *never* makes any sense. It never makes rational sense to do things that cause you or the people around you unnecessary pain. But addictive dynamics concoct justifications and delusions that somehow make such behavior seem reasonable, or even necessary.

Your belief system, for example, may be that people always take advantage of you and are abusive towards you. Part of you must know that the reason so many people have been abusive towards you is that you've chosen to get into relationships with abusive people and then tolerated their abuse. You've *picked* abusive people to be involved with! Part of you *wants* to be with abusive people, and that part of you –

which isn't really part of *you* at all – is your false self, your addiction persona.

Dysfunctional belief systems also have a nasty way of reinforcing themselves. If, for instance, you have the belief that people don't like you, that they are always mean and unfair to you, this belief is likely to make you hurt, angry, resentful, and anti-social. Human beings have a natural biological tendency upon seeing another human being who looks angry to be very wary of that person. Our evolutionary heritage, acting through our genes and our behavioral tendencies, unconsciously informs us that people who are very angry are also potentially danger-ous. So people who show up in the world as angry because they think everyone is always mean or indifferent to them, are very likely to be met with a certain hostility and indifference from other people, thus reinforcing the initial belief. It becomes another addictive loop.

But perhaps the most tragic, and more hidden, effect of dysfunc-tional belief systems is that they never allow us to truly live. The fears our belief systems have been constructed to shield us from will rarely lead to as much damage, will rarely cause us as much pain, as *not living*. Destructive world-views cause us profound pain in part because they don't allow us to fulfill our potential, to live the kind of life we're meant to live. And the sad truth is that most people in the modern world don't really live. As the psychologist Alfred Adler said of one such person: "To the question 'What use are you making of your talents?' he answers, 'This thing stops me; I cannot go ahead,' and points to his self-erected barricade."

A barricade of this type is constructed from a dysfunctional belief system. When our belief systems are dysfunctional, we typically don't want to take accountability for what's wrong with the choices we've been making, but instead want to blame other people or other circumstances for our plight – our parents, friends, co-workers, or just the cruel world in general. In other words, we feel like *victims*. Feeling like a victim probably typically comes from early childhood trauma, whether that trauma is severe or more subtle. When you're trauma-tized, you feel *victimized*, you feel like a victim. Then being a victim can become your story – you have the energy and posture of a victim, which will often lead to further victimization. Victimhood becomes your story and your life becomes about living that story.

When we have dysfunctional belief systems, there's an unconscious drive within us to reinforce our view of the world by having experiences that *confirm* that dysfunctional belief system. This at least gives us a false sense of security, an illusory feeling of safety, because it confirms our rightness about how the world operates. Our feeling of rightness gives a false sense of safety that is a dysfunctional attempt to combat a nearly constant state of survival mode. In a broad sense, this is the work of the addiction persona – if the addiction persona can keep you stuck in your dysfunctional belief system, the dysfunctional payoffs will continue in full force. If you believe that people just don't like you, then the addiction persona will "try" to reinforce that belief by keeping you stuck. The more stuck you are in that dysfunctional belief system, the more dysfunctional payoffs you'll receive from pain and distress, and the further out of balance you'll be. And the more out of balance you are, the more you'll be driven into the dysfunctional behavior that reinforces the belief system that keeps you stuck.

Another reason we can become so entrenched in and committed to our belief system is that we can easily confuse our belief system with our *self*. There's an illusion that if we jettison our dysfunctional belief systems we'll somehow lose part of ourselves. But a good portion of our belief systems very often have nothing to do with us – they're a consequence of early, often dysfunctional, childhood circumstances we had little or no control over. We typically absorb these belief systems from our parents and from the prevailing culture that we're born into.

If part of our belief system is clearly hurting us, however, we have to see that it's dysfunctional, and that we need to replace it with a belief system that's more aligned with the truth. A belief system that is based on the truth will always be functional, or homeostatic. And since our behavior will usually align with our belief system, if our belief systems are homeostatic, our behavior will be homeostatic also, and consequently we ourselves will generally be homeostatic.

The dysfunctional part of us fears that if even part of our false belief system is found to be incorrect, then everything about our lives would fall apart. And in a sense that's true. If your belief system is dysfunctional, that means it comes from the false self. And if the false part of your belief system is revealed as false, then part of your false self, your addiction persona, *will* start to crumble. The addiction persona, through the power of survival mode-driven drug payoffs, creates the illusion that it *is* your self, and that if you lose part of it, you'll be losing part of yourself. Moreover, the addiction persona tricks you into feeling that if you consistently made your way out of the survival-mode state that it keeps throwing you into, your survival would be severely threatened.

Despite the power of this illusion, however, it's quite the opposite of the truth. The addiction persona responds to *illusory* survival risks by throwing you into unnecessary, *dysfunctional* states of survival mode. The addiction persona obstructs, distorts, and disguises the real you, disguises your True Self. It takes a part of your True Self and spins a web of illusion around it loosely glued together with lies and false justifications. But if you can see through that tissue of lies, the web will begin to fray and finally disintegrate completely, uncovering the True Self.

Substance abusers typically provide us with the clearest examples of how addictive patterns operate. And substance abusers tend to be very inflammatory when you question their belief systems. Since that belief system is supporting the use of the drug that they're addicted to, they have all of their justifications firmly in place. But their whole belief system is a house of cards. If any part of that belief system is found to be wrong or nonsensical, the whole thing could collapse. Part of them actually believes those lies, but another part of them sees the truth. The addiction persona wants the drug and the True Self wants truth and homeostasis. Without their false belief systems, addicts know that they'll have to give up their drug. And the addiction persona wants to hold on to that drug.

Feeling and being "less than" is also a key part of the belief system of any substance abuser, although those feelings may be hidden beneath various "less than" compensations. Substance abusers, like all addicts, usually just don't know themselves, or have a remarkably distorted view of themselves – they may be truly unaware of their talents, for example, or they may know vaguely about those talents but diminish their importance. The more severe the addiction – whether it's an emotional, behavioral, or substance addiction – the greater the sense of "less than" and the more extreme the disconnection from self tends to be.

The false belief system that underlies any addiction ultimately exists only to justify the use of the drug that the addiction supplies. But when you question someone's belief system, especially someone who's deeply immersed in their addictions, from their perspective you're questioning who they *are*. It's the very foundation on which they stand, so when you threaten their belief system, they instinctually feel that you're threatening their very existence. Of course, this is just another illusion. People's belief systems can shift dramatically, but their bodies and minds hardly crumble into dust after these shifts. On the contrary, because such big shifts typically move people closer to the truth, the opposite will often happen – they'll typically become stronger physically and emotionally, and more at peace. The truth always seeks you out, and if you can loosen the grip of addiction, at some point the truth will find you.

The common notion, even among medical professionals, that drug addiction is an essentially incurable genetic "disease" is another example of a dysfunctional belief system. Based on the evidence, it's undeniable that some people are more genetically vulnerable to falling into various kinds of addictions than other people. And there is no doubt that addiction is at least a "syndrome," in that substantial, and often dramatic, changes occur in the brain of a substance abuser or alcoholic – although, at least for the most part, those changes are likely to be reversible in most cases. Calling addiction a "disease," however, is, at best, profoundly misleading. When we hear the word "disease" the image that's conjured in our minds is of a condition that we cannot escape, but can only treat and manage, a condition that is chronic, and that will probably kill us prematurely. And this image doesn't really fit what addiction is.

The movement that initially led to labeling addiction a "disease" was entirely well-meaning. It sought to take the stigma away from substance abusers and alcoholics, so that they wouldn't be "blamed" for their condition and so that their addictions wouldn't be viewed as moral failings. But if you take the attitude, as we do in this book, that all addicts, all people, only act destructively to themselves and to others because they are wholly or largely unconscious of addictive dynamics, that they are driven into their addiction out of an illusory and irrational survival fear, you won't blame them anyway.

Although calling addiction a "disease" had the well-meaning intention of trying to help substance abusers and alcoholics, it has actually ended up profoundly *hurting* them. Because viewing your addiction as an incurable disease creates a false belief that only serves to reinforce the addiction. There is probably no single factor more likely to keep substance abusers stuck in their addiction than convincing them that their addiction is a disease that they are genetically doomed to suffer, with the supposed weight of scientific evidence supporting this highly dubious claim. The claim provides substance abusers with a powerful justification for continuing the addiction. It creates a dysfunctional belief system.

Do drug addiction, alcoholism, or compulsive gambling, for example, qualify as genetic "diseases"? Many medical professionals would claim that they do. But the scientific evidence does not in any way support this claim. Our view is that addiction is *never* a natural phenomenon, or at least is extremely rare. There is no precedent in our genetic or hunter-gatherer heritage for our being substance abusers or alcoholics – the phenomenon is purely a consequence of radically unnatural modern environments. It's true that in certain unnatural environments, some people will be more prone to becoming alcoholics than other people because of their genetic vulnerabilities. But if those people were raised in hunter-gatherer bands, *none* of them would become alcoholics. Many nomadic hunter-gatherers in their natural state have access to alcoholic and narcotic substances – but there's little or no evidence that they ever become *addicted* to those substances.

When previously nomadic groups became sedentary and shifted to the agricultural lifestyle, however, addiction of many types became common. But that's because the *environment* changed into one that human beings are not well-equipped biologically to deal with. If there's little or no addiction when we live in the natural state for which we're biologically adapted, it makes no sense to talk about "addiction genes." Rather, versions of genes exist that make us more susceptible to addiction only when we live in unnatural environments, and particularly when we have unnaturally traumatic upbringings.

Does nicotine addiction qualify as a "disease?" Many studies have shown that nicotine addiction is one of the most difficult substance addictions to overcome. But if nicotine addiction is a "disease," it is a disease that millions of people have cured themselves of by quitting smoking, often without the help of any specific program or therapy. And although many people who have quit smoking, even for good, continue to have cravings for cigarettes, many others do not. Something in their minds shifted, sometimes in response to some dramatic life event or sudden revelation, and they just decided that they weren't going to smoke anymore. People can, and millions of people have, quit substance addictions simply by making the choice not to use the substance anymore, and by continuing to abide by that decision.

The same cannot be said, however, of neurological diseases like Alzheimer's or Parkinson's Disease. People with Alzheimer's can't simply make a behavioral decision and be "cured" of their disease. And so it's very misleading to equate substance abuse to true diseases like Alzheimer's or Parkinson's. That doesn't at all mean that overcoming addiction is easy, of course, or that the millions of people who have tried unsuccessfully to overcome their substance addictions are lesser people in any way. But falsely viewing their addictions as "diseases" only makes it more difficult for them to overcome the addictions that cause them so much pain.

To give another illustration of the widespread fallacy that leads people to view addiction as a "disease," consider the case of diabetes. Anthropologists have found little or no evidence for *any* kind of diabetes among hunter-gatherers. Type I, or juvenile, diabetes appears to result from an autoimmune disorder. Autoimmune disorders are probably largely triggered by a number of unnatural aspects of modern life, many of which, such as chronically high stress levels, appear to be driven and sustained by addictive dynamics. Type II diabetes seems to be almost solely a consequence of unnatural modern diets, particularly diets rich in refined carbohydrates such as white flour and processed sugar, which are profoundly unnatural substances for a human being to consume. Hunter-gatherers eating their natural diets of nuts, fruits, roots, vegetables, and lean game animals will very rarely, if ever, develop diabetes.

But if you took a hundred hunter-gatherers and forced them to eat a lot of fast food, donuts, and gummy bears for a year, a substantial proportion of them – perhaps about half – would probably develop diabetes. Does that mean that these fifty or so hunter-gatherers have genes "for" diabetes? Not at all. They have genes that make them more susceptible to diabetes *only when they eat a radically unnatural diet.* Similarly, people do not have genes "for" addiction – but living in the unnatural circumstances of the modern world, some people become significantly more at risk than others for developing various addictions. And just as most people living in industrialized cultures have the power to *choose* to eat healthy diets, they have the power to stop their substance addictions. Admittedly, modern culture aids and abets all types of addiction at almost every turn. But that's very different from saying that certain people have genes that doom them to lives of substance abuse or overeating. It's a critical distinction.

If you believe and appreciate the central premise of this book, you can see that nearly all of us, quite literally, are addicts. And part of every addict *knows* the truth. Part of every addict knows that he or she has the power to *choose*. Part of you knows that you have the capacity to choose not to overeat, drink excessively, or otherwise cause yourself unnecessary pain. Part of you also knows that your life can be very different from what it is if you simply make different choices.

Part of you knows that the justifications and excuses you use for your own addictive patterns and self-defeating behaviors make no sense at all. Self-defeating behavior never makes any rational sense. But if you stopped telling yourself that same dysfunctional story, you could no longer justify all the unhealthy patterns you find yourself slipping into. If you let go of your story, you would have to let go of all the excuses you've been using that have allowed you to keep taking your drugs. But understand that if something is obviously wrong in your life, then something you mistakenly believe to be true about yourself is probably hurting you. If you can align your belief system with the truth and with homeostasis, your behavior will follow, and you will move closer to the True Self.

CHAPTER 10

TAKING ACCOUNTABILITY

The underlying reality of all human behavior is that we do whatever we do, either consciously or unconsciously, to get a bio-chemical payoff in our brains. That's simply the way we're put together as biological organisms. We may get those payoffs in healthy ways or unhealthy ways, but if we didn't get *some* sort of payoff from what we did, we wouldn't do it.

Even when we think we're acting unselfishly, "out of the goodness of our hearts," the core reason we're acting the way we are is that *we're* getting some sort of payoff from those actions. Fortunately, it often does feel very good to do generous things for other people. Studies have shown, for example, that giving money to charitable organizations strongly activates reward centers in the brain and probably leads to substantial releases of endorphin. So whatever we choose to do will give us some sort of biochemical payoff. We're simply healthiest when both the payoffs and what we're doing to receive the payoffs are homeostatic.

Nothing is more homeostatic than authentic love, and authentic love will always lead us towards homeostasis. But it may be easier than you think to deceive yourself about love. You may do something, apparently selflessly, for other people, and, although it makes a good story to tell to yourself and others that you're doing it out of love, the truth might be that you're getting a substantial payoff – a dysfunctional payoff – from being a "martyr," for example, rather than a functional payoff from helping another human being out of love. If you're clearly resenting what you're doing, or are angry because the other person seems ungrateful – then you're doing what you're doing, at least in part, to derive a dysfunctional payoff. You're doing it because *you,* for whatever reason, don't feel okay about yourself unless you're the person who gives and gives, even if the person you're giving too is ungrateful. Although it may seem like you're doing something good, something unselfish, you're actually feeding the addictive drive. If you can get yourself back into balance, maybe you would do exactly the same thing for someone truly out of love, and not resent it or feel martyred by it. Then you would be serving and aligning with the homeostatic drive. But if your self-image continually reinforces how "unselfish" you are, it's very likely that you're disconnected from your true motivation for doing what you do.

People who are overly invested in their self-image in this way also often have the tendency to "judge" other people. "Judging" someone, in this sense, means making that other person "less than" or "more than" you. But there's an important distinction between "judging" and "assessing." When you make an "assessment," you're mainly trying to *understand*. What are the relevant features of other people's circumstances, belief systems, and life history that might motivate them to act the way that they act? When you make such an assessment, it's perfectly reasonable, appropriate, and healthy to disapprove of someone's *behavior* if that behavior doesn't align with your own values. Then you're disapproving of the behavior, but you're not judging the *person* – you're not making them "less than" you, you're not looking down on them, just because they did something you disapprove of. You're not making their worth as a human being any less than yours just because your interpretation of what they said or did doesn't align with your own views and beliefs.

Remember that people's behavior can improve, sometimes dramatically, within a relatively short period. And presumably during that period their intrinsic, potential worth won't have changed at all. So while people always need to be held accountable for what they do, just because they do bad things doesn't make them bad people. None of us is in a position to judge another person's intrinsic worth, since we can't know who they truly are or what they're capable of. Perhaps God can make that kind of judgment, but no human being can.

Nevertheless, it can give people quite a "charge," quite a rush, to judge other people, to make those people "less than." In almost every case, people who are always trying to make other people "less than" are themselves compensating for their own feelings of "less than."

Judgment, however, is clearly a *dysfunctional* attempt to elevate your status. Why is it dysfunctional? Because by making someone "less than" you're making yourself "more than," and neither standpoint is homeostatic. On the pendulum of non-homeostasis, feeling "more than" is equivalent to a stimulant, and feeling "less than" is equivalent to a depressant. If you consistently feel one, at some point you're going to swing over and feel the other. Whenever you're using any thought or behavior to make yourself feel "less than" or "more than" someone else, you're using that behavior or thought as a drug.

When we make other people "more than" ourselves, when we put them "up on a pedestal," we're making *ourselves* "less than," and that's never healthy either. Other people may *do* very commendable things, they may behave admirably, but that doesn't necessarily make their intrinsic worth as human beings greater than anyone else's. Elevating other people to this exalted position creates an imbalance in us. So then, at some point – because it turns out that it feels unpleasant to consistently have someone else be "more" than us – we'll probably want to knock them down from that pedestal and make *them* "less than." This is part of the celebrity culture that drives so much of the popular media. We make celebrities "more than" us, and then, when they slip up, when they stumble, we take a sadistic delight in making fun of them, in kicking them when they're down, in making them "less than."

Some people who commendably try to avoid this tendency become so concerned about the "prohibition" against judgment that they overcompensate and feel it's also wrong to make *assessments* about what other people do or how they act. But we can't help assessing everything in our surroundings. We must have *some* response to what we see, hear, and feel about other people and what they do and say. There's nothing unhealthy about that as long as we're not ranking their worth as human beings.

The drug of looking down on people, of making them "less than," can certainly be seductive. But it will only send us out of balance. We may, by virtue of genetics, upbringing, knowledge, or higher consciousness, be so fortunate to be thought of as good, compassionate, kind, intelligent, attractive people. But that doesn't make our worth as human beings greater than anyone else's. Viewing all people as having equivalent worth is a homeostatic standpoint. It's stable and peaceful, probably because it aligns with the truth. Assess people's behavior, try to understand why they do what they do, but never judge them as human beings, because that will only feed addiction within *you*. Similarly, when something you do consistently feeds the sense that *you're* "less than," but you keep doing it anyway, that's a reliable tag for an addictive behavior.

You're not a bad person if you refuse to face your addictions. And unless you're caught for doing something criminal, or are killed or injured, no one can really stop you from engaging in addictive patterns if that's what you choose to do. The key point is that your addictions are always bad for *you*. Your addictions cause you pain, they diminish your life. Whatever successes and fulfilling moments you've had in your life, you would have far more, perhaps infinitely more, without your addictions. Though some addictions are more obvious than others, no addiction, however minor in its manifestation, is ever benign. A relatively small unbalancing effect from one addiction often enables and perpetuates other, more serious, addictions. Choose addiction if you want – but when you do so, know that you'll always be choosing pain.

Persistent pain, in turn, will almost always give rise to at least some anger. When wild animals or human hunter-gatherers are in physical or emotional pain, the painful feeling acts as a signal for an injury that poses a true survival risk. The feeling of anger often triggered by such pain will fuel bodily responses or actions that are designed to promote survival. In both animals and people, anger can therefore sometimes be entirely functional.

But if you're still angry with someone whom you were hurt by many months or years ago, that anger is almost certainly being driven by addiction now, and is no longer functional. When you're deep in your anger addiction alter, you can somehow always create a justification for the anger. A justification is hardly ever a *complete* lie, or something that is *completely* absurd. A good justification has to be based on something at least somewhat reasonable or else it simply wouldn't work as a justification.

True forgiveness would quickly extinguish all of your justifications for feeling anger. The addictive drive, therefore, doesn't want you to forgive any particular person because then you could no longer justify your anger. Then you would be taking your foot off of their throat and letting them off the hook. If you forgive them, you'll no longer be *right* about what awful bastards they are! But at some point – a point that comes sooner than you might think – your anger mainly serves to hurt *you*. That anger will keep you in a false and persistent state of jaw-clenching, blood-pressure-raising, psychologically-unbalancing survival mode, and so it will be terrible for your physical, emotional, and spiritual health.

When you've been hurt by someone, it's also natural to create an association between the person and your pain. An easy leap to make, then, is that the person is not only causing you pain, but is *responsible* for your pain, and probably *intended* to cause you pain. Then you've created a full-fledged projection onto that person that will justify your anger towards them. Most addictions wouldn't be able to supply their drug payoffs without such projections. But this projection is almost always an illusion, a lie. People rarely intend with full consciousness to cause other people unnecessary pain – they almost always do so out of their own ignorance, or out of their own state of survival mode. When we're in survival mode we "go unconscious" to at least some degree. In wild animals and hunter-gatherers, unconscious patterns, because they're fast and generally efficient, promote survival during emergency situations. But addiction misappropriates this biological tendency by using unconscious patterns that serve dysfunctional ends.

If you're still angry at someone for something that happened twenty years ago, or even twenty days ago, you have to take accountability for that anger. You may well fall into the illusion that your anger is *their* fault, but of course this is just another lie. *You're* the one who's angry. You're the one who should be making decisions that allow you to take care of yourself so that you don't experience any unnecessary pain. If other people have caused you so much pain, your responsibility to yourself is to make decisions – such as modifying your relationship, or perhaps cutting that person out of your life entirely – so that you will no longer experience that hurt. People just do what they do and what they do is never a reflection of your own intrinsic worth as a human being. Remember that and you'll always be able to forgive.

What you'll also often find is that if you can forgive one person, if you can stop feeling angry at them for how much they've hurt you, you'll soon become angry at someone else. The specific object of your obsessive anger isn't necessarily so important. A particular obsession can create the illusion of absolute importance, but that's usually only because it has temporarily become the dominant obsession among many potential obsessions. The current obsession is the one that has "won out" in the battle for your attention, and it temporarily becomes the dominant vehicle for an addictive payoff. The truth is that the *state of being angry itself* is what is giving you the addictive payoff that you keep going back for more of.

When you understand and appreciate that the vast majority of the time *you* are the one who's choosing anger, pain, and other distressing emotional states, you're ready to start taking full accountability for what you do and have done. If you can't take accountability for the negative, destructive things that you do, you won't be able to take accountability for the *positive* things you do either. People with chronically low self-esteem typically don't take full accountability for themselves, and so when they have some great success in their lives, they will often somehow feel that they didn't deserve that success, that they just got lucky, that they're still just as worthless as they've always been. But if you take full accountability for your failings, for your mistakes and destructive behavior, then you'll be able to take full accountability for your successes as well.

Another common addictive pattern is to repeatedly recall stupid or hurtful things you've said or done in the past. If these are things you've already reviewed and duly chastised yourself about, understand that there's only one reason you're calling up those memories: to get a drug payoff from the feelings of shame, regret, embarrassment, or guilt that the memories arouse in you. Recalling one of those distressing memories is like having someone whack you in the back of the head. What a nice, bracing charge!

If you're growing, changing, and maturing, almost by definition you'll be doing things differently now than you have in the past. So it's natural to regret certain things you did or said. It's a sign of growth. When we act out of addiction or ignorance, we typically do regrettable things. If you didn't do some things differently now than you would have done ten or twenty years ago, then you probably haven't grown very much as a person during that time, and that's not necessarily very healthy either. So having some regrets is natural, and not necessarily a bad thing. Feel that regret, accept it, and pass through it – just don't get addicted to it.

Addiction is also often responsible for creating "forbidden" thoughts in our minds that most people would be afraid or embarrassed to admit they have. These thoughts typically violate societal norms and may be sacrilegious, violent, sexually inappropriate, or potentially deeply hurtful to other people. The reason such thoughts can throw us into survival mode is probably that, if we were in a hunter-gatherer band, we would fear that if everyone knew we had such horrible, violent, sexually perverse, or destructive thoughts, it may lead to us being ostracized within the band, increasing our risk of not being able to find a mate, or of getting thrown out of the band entirely.

Some studies have suggested, for example, that at least one reason young mothers can develop obsessive-compulsive disorder (OCD), or even post-partum depression, is that they can't shake the obsessive thought of wanting to physically harm their babies. Such mothers typically feel horrible shame about the persistent thoughts. When hunter-gatherer mothers sense that, given their own current circumstances, the prospects for the survival of their newborn babies is low, they will often kill or abandon their babies. If our ancestors didn't have these kinds of urges in certain survival-related circum- stances, they never would have survived and bequeathed to us their genes. But in most cases in modern life, the obsessive thoughts in a young mother about harming her baby probably come, either directly or indirectly, from addiction. If a new mother is constantly in survival mode due to her own neuroses – due to an anxiety disorder, for example – that constant state of survival mode may trigger the ancient biological urge to kill or abandon the baby. Since the repetition of obsessive thoughts about harming the baby will further feed and reinforce addiction, it becomes yet another cyclical, addictive loop.

The pain of young mothers caught in such an addictive loop is typically severe. But if they can see that this loop is probably the work of the addiction persona – that, in a real sense, those impulses don't come from *them* at all – they can see through the illusions that are driving that loop, and extinguish the whole pattern. Similarly, the vast majority of unspeakable thoughts any of us have don't, in effect, come from *us*, and are not a true reflection of who we are as human beings. They typically arise in the mind to feed addiction, to supply a drug. When you're in a state of flow, of homeostasis, these forbidden thoughts will almost never arise. And if they did, you would probably laugh at them rather than be disturbed by them. It would be different if the unspeakable thoughts led to unspeakable *actions*. But they're just *thoughts*.

These thoughts will mainly arise, and have their jarring effects, when we're out of balance, when we're struggling, and the brain falls into survival mode. When you begin to see the true genesis and purpose of most of these thoughts, you may never have them again, and, if you do, you won't take them so seriously. If you don't take them seriously, they won't supply much of a payoff, and the neural networks that drive them will become weaker and will be less likely to generate those thoughts in the first place.

Because we get payoffs from being in both homeostasis and non-homeostasis, from being in a state of "flow" or being in survival mode, the two states can compete, in a sense, to pull us towards them. Ideally, we would spend most of our time in a state of flow, an almost pure state of homeostasis in which we feel completely alive and are completely absorbed in what we're doing. In a state of flow, our cup runneth over – we have no needs, no wants, no fears. We just *are* – we're *being*, we're alive and vital and doing whatever it is that we're driven to do in that moment. Biochemically, our dopamine and endorphin levels are probably just about optimal – they're perfectly balanced, not too low and not too high. In a state of flow, the thought of being actively angry at someone who hurt us five or fifteen years ago seems completely absurd – and it *is* absurd. In a state of flow, the addictive drive has no power over us. When we're in a state of flow, addiction and survival mode seem far, far away.

The illusion created by addiction is that our survival is at significant risk in the short term, which it very rarely is. But of course in the long term the truth is that we're all going to die. To not face the reality of death squarely is to create a division within ourselves that will only feed addiction. When we have integrated within ourselves the knowledge that at some point we're going to die, we can see the absurdity of obsessing about or focusing on things that, in reality, hold little importance for us. The acceptance of death sets life into clearer relief. It's much more difficult for addiction to sabotage our lives with its fraudulent death threats when we've fully accepted that the real thing will be here eventually anyway. The more we can reinforce the truth about any aspect of our lives, or of life in general, the more we will dissolve addiction. The truth settles, relaxes, and ultimately liberates us, because it always leads away from addiction and towards homeostasis.

CHAPTER 11

INTERVENTION AND SPONTANEOUS RECOVERY

A woman we know whom we'll call Julie had an intervention many years ago. Julie was, and still is, a nurse. She began smoking cigarettes when she was a teenager. In her early twenties Julie had her first son, Robert. She tried to stop smoking several times during this period, but she just couldn't, and although she felt horrible about it, she continued to smoke cigarettes while she was pregnant. A few years later, she had her second son, Kyle, and also continued to smoke while she was pregnant with him. When Kyle was a baby, Julie would often leave him in his crib while she snuck outside for a quick smoke. One day, when Kyle was about seventeen months old, Julie put him in his crib in the living room with a few toys and walked out to her backyard to smoke a cigarette. When she walked back in her house and looked into the living room, she saw that Kyle had somehow gotten out of his crib and was now sitting on the floor with a plastic bag over his head.

Julie rushed over to Kyle and pulled the bag from his head. Although Kyle's face had literally turned purple, to Julie's profound relief, he was okay. After the pallor of his skin had returned to normal, she put Kyle back in his crib. Then she grabbed the pack of cigarettes she had in her purse, tore the pack in half, and threw the whole thing in the garbage. Kyle is now in his mid-twenties, and Julie says that since that day, she never once smoked or even craved a cigarette. In fact, when she saw other people smoking, especially for the first few years after Kyle's plastic bag incident, she would often become physically ill.

Millions of people have similar stories of events – we call them "life interventions" – that caused them to give up destructive and dangerous addictions. Because this happens so frequently, you can see why it's misleading to call addiction a "disease." If people have a good enough reason to quit *any* addiction, or if something happens to them that allows them to really *see*, to really *get*, how destructive their addictions are to themselves and to the people around them, they will quit those addictions and never look back. The majority of people just don't have an intervention quite as powerful or effective as Julie's, so they continue justifying and engaging in their addictions. Although Julie could somehow justify continuing to smoke during her pregnancies – even though, as a trained nurse, she knew quite well how unhealthy that was for her babies – those justifications and excuses simply couldn't survive after the day she found Kyle with a plastic bag over his head. Those justifications would never work for her anymore. She saw the truth of what her addiction was doing to her and her children, and thereafter she would never be able to *un*-see that truth. When a profound truth reveals itself to you with such force and clarity, you never forget it.

Many people require some sort of intervention to quit their addictions. This can be a life intervention, like it was with Julie. A life intervention is an event or circumstance that occurs during the course of everyday life that is potentially life-altering. Interventions can also be "staged." A professional interventionist, for example, may gather the friends and family of a substance abuser and directly confront him about all the pain the addiction is causing both him and the people who care about him. Other interventions are more subtle – they can be created by new information that suddenly causes people to see the world and their lives in a different way, that somehow illuminates their situation. It is our fervent hope that this book will act as such an intervention for anyone who reads it.

Any addictive pattern is encoded within and driven by a neural network that acts as an "alter." That neural network is in turn part of a larger network responsible for the addiction persona as a whole. An intervention, especially a powerful intervention, creates a new associative network that becomes woven into the old neural network responsible for the addiction alter. In a sense, such an intervention acts as a "reverse trauma" that can at least partially undo the effects of the childhood traumas that often create particular addictive patterns. Thereafter, whenever the old addiction alter that's responsible for that addictive pattern is triggered, the memories and feelings associated with the intervention will also quickly be triggered.

In Julie's case, anything that reminded her of cigarettes quickly reminded her of how her cigarette addiction almost killed her son.

And so the new neural network never allowed the old addiction alter to be sufficiently activated to produce even a craving for cigarettes. As the days, weeks, and months went by without the old addiction alter being triggered, the neural network that drove that alter became progressively weaker, until this network may have disappeared altogether, with perhaps only a vague residue remaining in the brain. The intervention, or reverse trauma, that Julie experienced, where her addiction-driven behavior almost led to the death of her son, was far more powerful than her cigarette addiction itself, and so that trauma began to dissolve her addiction almost immediately. Any intervention, even a more subtle one, similarly has the power to dissolve *any* addiction, whether it is an emotional, behavioral, or substance addiction.

Life interventions have the greatest chance of creating a spontaneous recovery from an addiction if the intervention directly impacts a critical core value for the person. Although Julie wasn't always an ideal mother, she tried her best to be the best possible mother she could be, given her circumstances and personal issues, and she listed "being a good mother" as her number one core value. Typically, when people clearly begin to see how their addictions impact their most dearly held core values – and addictions always *do* impact those core values – they'll be ready to overcome those addictions.

Julie's primary intervention, fortunately, resulted in no serious damage to either her or to Kyle. Other interventions can be far more painful and can't necessarily be rectified so easily. But it usually isn't in any way a rationalization to think of even the most painful interventions as true gifts. There is always something profound to be gained from a life intervention. Life interventions almost always happen because of some imbalance in the way you've been living, the way you've been approaching your life. It's possible the intervention is just something random that happened that has no real bearing on your situation or the choices you've been making. But that's very unlikely.

Most life interventions are *telling you something*: they identify things you're doing, decisions you're making that are not aligned with the truth of who you are and what your deepest intentions are. When something very painful happens to you, try to think about which of your addictions the intervention might be addressing and which out-of-balance aspects of your belief system or general orientation it might be illuminating. This is what the intervention, at least in part, is "meant" to be a correction to. What is the intervention trying to get you to see?

As painful as interventions usually are, if you can accept what a particular intervention is trying to get you to confront, in all likelihood you'll eventually be truly grateful for it. It's simply a law of nature that persistent addictive patterns will eventually lead to life interventions. And such interventions can give you the gift of breaking through one or more of your addictions. Overcoming an addiction doesn't need to involve any pain at all – but, in practice, it often does. To overcome our addictions, to rectify belief systems or tendencies that have become out of balance, most of us seem to need a slap in the face that really stings. If you don't respond to the slap, understand that the next blow you absorb, the next intervention, will probably be even more painful – it will be a closed fist or an elbow to your face or your gut. Listen to your interventions. If you don't listen to the first or second intervention, they're going to keep coming, and you'll soon be hobbling around with dents all over your body and your spirit.

Any challenge, any difficult period we go through, can act as an intervention and truly facilitate our growth and healing. Very often, situations arise that draw us back into our addictive patterns. But typically we ourselves have at least partially, and usually unconsciously, created or contributed to those circumstances. Such circumstances can shine a clear and powerful light on our patterns and tendencies if we take full accountability for what we do and resist the temptation to blame other people for whatever difficulties we experience. If we use personal challenges as opportunities to identify, address, and overcome our addictions, we can truly come to see those challenges as great gifts that helped us move closer to a full realization of the True Self.

A certain amount of pain and loss is inevitable, of course, and sometimes it's difficult to know why certain things happen. But every life intervention, almost without exception, can be used as an opportunity for growth, and every life intervention will help you to grow and ultimately to heal if you feel it, process it, and try to understand it. Even the most painful events and circumstances can often be passed through relatively quickly if you don't allow yourself to become *addicted* to the pain, but still allow yourself to *feel* and process the pain.

When something very painful happens, it does force you to *feel*. Feeling, in that moment, is inescapable. So a painful event or loss can become an opportunity to feel emotions more authentically, to return to the ground of feeling. Some people create a non-homeostatic, addiction-enabling disconnection within themselves by not facing and feeling their authentic pain, by repressing it; and other people use any pain they feel or experience as a drug that can be recollected and re-engaged in whenever they need a jolt of dopamine and endorphin. Achieving the proper balance between these two extremes is the key to healing.

Although striking this balance may seem tricky, remember that we have a guide and sensor within us that is specifically designed for this purpose: homeostasis. The homeostatic drive is an almost magical capacity we all have within us that strives to bring us back into balance after we become distressed, to make things right with us, to allow us to live the life we're meant to live. When you connect to your homeostatic drive, that drive will *automatically*, just by its intrinsic nature, allow you to find the balance between those extremes.

Even now, Julie could be filled with shame that her son almost died because of her addiction-driven negligence. Or she could be wallowing in regret that she perhaps permanently damaged Kyle's physical and emotional health by continuing to smoke while she was pregnant with him. But there's nothing to be done about that now. We can only do the best we can *now*, in the present. The most important thing about any life intervention is that, once it has passed, it has to be accepted. Maybe it can be healed or repaired, and maybe not; maybe its repercussions are major and maybe they're minor. It may alter your future decisions overtly, subtly, or not at all. But it has to be accepted. It *is*. Part of getting addicted to a past trauma is the illusion that if you obsess about it enough, if you feel the pain of the trauma over and over, that somehow you can change it, make it different. But the trauma has to be faced and somehow integrated into your psyche. And then you have to choose to focus on how you live *now*, the choices you're making *now*.

It's often said that the "universe" somehow confronts us with what we need to deal with to grow emotionally and spiritually. This may well be true, and the addiction dynamic could at least partially explain it. We find ourselves in certain situations or with certain people because those situations and those people feed into our addictions, and therefore supply us with a drug. But if we're going to grow, we need to overcome those addictions. If we continue to use those circumstances as a drug, we'll just continue to remain stuck in our addictive patterns. And then perhaps the increasing severity of those addictive patterns will lead to a life intervention that will finally slap us in the face hard enough to wake us up.

You don't need to wait for something horrible or painful to happen for you to address and overcome your addictions. Admittedly, for the majority of people, the process of overcoming addictive patterns often takes continuous work, numerous interventions, and various types of reinforcement over an extended period. But it doesn't have to. If you can see the dynamics of addiction clearly, if you can just tell yourself the truth about what you're doing and why you're doing it, and fully commit to that truth, you can simply *choose* to pass through any addiction right now.

CHAPTER 12

Triggers and "Neural Antibodies"

Perhaps the most important part of beating addiction is identifying and recognizing the triggers that send you hurtling into your addictive patterns. It can be little things. Maybe when you're meeting someone and they're late, it triggers you into feeling "less than," or into becoming extremely angry. It's easy to justify feeling that way – it's their fault for being late! – but ultimately feeling "less than" and unreasonably angry only hurts *you*. If someone else is late, it isn't a reflection of your own worth. The initial hint of anger may give you an indication of what decisions might be best for you in the future – perhaps you won't choose to meet that person again under those circumstances, or perhaps under any circumstance at all. But engaging in that feeling of anger for more than a few moments doesn't make any sense, because it's only hurting *you*. If you want to feel less pain and distress and live more fully, you'll have to learn to beat triggers like that.

You can think of the process that leads to the full-blown triggering of an addictive pattern as a series of dominoes. The first domino that falls is the trigger. If nothing interferes, the momentum of that first domino will eventually activate the entire addictive sequence, with a big, juicy drug payoff at the end. If your friend is late, you may, for example, start to think of several occasions when you felt painfully "less than." Yes, in fact this very friend who is late has often made you feel "less than!" Because that's how she looks at you. She looks down at you, she laughs at you behind your back, she doesn't care about you. Those thoughts, whether or not they're based in reality, are the sound of the dominoes falling.

Even once you've mastered your addiction, it can be very difficult to keep that first domino from toppling over. The trick is to keep the first domino from crashing into the next domino in the sequence, which would then initiate the whole violent, painful, self-destructive chain reaction. If you can learn to mute that trigger, if you can quickly become aware of that first tottering domino, you can catch it and safely remove it. You're not "less than;" you're not angry. Someone is just late. It's no reflection whatsoever on you as a person. It's about them, it's not about you. Your feelings of self-worth will be unaffected by their being late. You don't feel *good* about it – but you don't feel "less than" either, and you don't feel especially angry. They're just not always good about being on time. Maybe you won't choose to meet up somewhere with them again. But what they do has nothing to do with your worth as a person.

Imagine you're a fish in a lake and fishermen are dropping their lines into the water trying to catch you. The worms they dangle to tempt you are the triggers for your addictions. You see a nice juicy worm and you can't resist – you bite into it, and wham! There's a hook in this worm! There's a jolt of pain, and then the fisherman reels you into his boat with the hook still sticking painfully in your mouth. He finally removes the hook and, since you're beneath the commercial size limit, mercifully throws you back in the water, with your mouth still bleeding. That's the full-blown addictive sequence, when all the dominoes fall. Your addiction may or may not lead to your being gutted and filleted, but it will always cause you pain, sometimes enormous pain.

Once your mouth heals, you start looking around the lake again. The fishermen are having a lot of success with fish like you, and so they tell their friends: "Hey, the fish are really biting here!" And so now there are even more worms in the water than there were before. Part of you knows there are hooks inside those worms, but another part of you doesn't quite want to accept it. Because those worms look so good! You see a particularly nice one, and you bite into it. Part of you knew there was a hook inside the worm, but you didn't listen to yourself. And it turns out that biting into the hook still really, really hurts. The fisherman reels you in, takes the hook out of your mouth again and throws you back in the water.

After several weeks, your mouth is finally healed, and you look around the lake. This time you know, you really know about the worms and the hooks. You understand how it all works – you get it. You're not going to bite on those worms, you're going to eat something else, something that won't involve any pain so you won't have to spend all those weeks with an aching mouth. And then when you start refusing to bite on the fishermen's worms, guess what? The fishermen pull their lines out of the water, row back to shore, and try their luck in another lake. When you commit to not being hooked by your triggers anymore, those triggers will show up in your life less and less frequently.

When you allow your addictions to be triggered, those triggers, or hooks, will just show up because part of you *wants* them to show up. You'll unconsciously create circumstances and make choices that present you with the very triggers that lead into your painful, distressing addictive patterns. But if you stop biting on those hooks, if you're determined not to be triggered anymore, fewer of those triggers will show up – because now you're more conscious of how your addictive patterns operate.

If you want to overcome all of your addictions, you would ideally want to identify not only all of your addictive patterns, but also all of the triggers that trigger you into those patterns. But remember that your addiction alters are all linked together in a web, a network, and so if you disrupt one addictive pattern, that will also disrupt a number of other related patterns. Furthermore, changing dysfunctional, underlying *belief systems* about yourself can almost instantly disrupt nearly all of your addictions.

Once you've identified some of your addictive patterns, you can begin to form what we call "neural antibodies" for those patterns. Typically, a neural antibody is a thought pattern that reinforces the *truth* about your circumstances, because the false self, being fundamentally irrational, can only be sustained by lies and illusions. An effective neural antibody also taps into deeply-felt emotions that would make it clear just how much pain your addictive behavior or destructive thought pattern is causing you. When an entire suite of neural antibodies is consistently mobilized, the neural networks responsible for addictive patterns will no longer be activated. The once deeply-ingrained addictive networks will therefore become progressively weaker, and may disappear altogether, while new, healthier networks will become progressively stronger.

In the immune system, antibodies identify and then facilitate the destruction of pathogens that try to invade your body. Just as many different types of molecules – such as T cells, B cells, and phagocytes

– are necessary to combat invading viruses or bacteria, it's often necessary to mobilize several different types of neural antibodies to destroy or inactivate a trigger for one or more of your addictions. The same neural antibodies that inactivate triggers can also be used once the entire addiction neural network has been activated – but it's far preferable to inactivate the actual trigger, because then the neural antibody will keep the addiction alter from being activated in the first place. In the same sense, it's much better for the immune system to destroy and eliminate a flu virus before it actually gives you the flu.

In the immune system, once antibodies to specific viruses are created, they remain for a lifetime, without any additional work on your part. One extra requirement with neural antibodies, however, is that, at least at first, they require *consciousness* for them to be efficiently mobilized. You have to stay aware so that you know when you're slipping back into old addictive patterns, or when you might be generating new addictive patterns. Your neural antibodies will protect you from addiction, but they require your consciousness, they need you to be at least partially "awake" so that they can do their work.

Enhanced consciousness, however, should never be confused with self-consciousness. Self-consciousness comes from a feeling of "less than." When you're self-conscious, you're anxious that people will perceive you or judge you unfavorably, thus causing your status to drop. You may over-compensate by acting "more than," but that compensation is only driven by underlying feelings of "less than." Consciousness is just being aware of your self and your environment, and, in particular, being aware of your old dysfunctional patterns so that you can avoid slipping back into them. Consciousness is being aware of what you do and why you do it. The fear of judgment actually reduces consciousness because when you project onto other people that they are judging you, usually fearing that they will judge you unfavorably, your attention and awareness will become distracted and split.

Addiction is not in any way out to get you – it simply happens when your brain gets tricked into going into survival mode inappropriately. But once you can assure the addiction persona that things are safe, that your survival *is not* at risk, it will stop triggering you into survival mode. It *never* makes any sense to be triggered into an addictive pattern, and becoming triggered is incompatible with the truth.

The reason you're getting triggered is that you're falling into an illusion – you're getting triggered because, in effect, you're unconsciously *choosing* pain and justifying that choice with lies you're telling to yourself. A team of neural antibodies will attack that lie from every angle.

You may, for instance, be stagnating in continual feelings of resentment or anger towards someone you were hurt by. Part of you doesn't *want* to forgive that person because, if you do forgive them, you'll have to give up the drug of anger, of victimhood. Your neural antibodies in this circumstance might include: reinforcing that your continued anger is hurting *you*; that the person must have acted out of unconsciousness, fear, or pain; that you're only going back to your hurt and anger to get a drug payoff; that what other people do has nothing to do with your own worth, which is infinite. You may choose several other neural antibodies to mobilize, hopefully some or all of which have a strong emotional resonance for you. Typically the last neural antibody to have in the sequence is one that counsels and reminds you: come back into the present, the Now. Because real life is always in the Now, in homeostasis, and in "flow."

If you know that the patterns you're falling into are addictions, but you still can't shake them, then you either need more neural antibodies, or you need to strengthen and reinforce the neural anti-bodies you've already created. Just as you learn how to play the piano by repetition, by reinforcement, your neural antibodies need to be reinforced and repeatedly used, at least at first, so that they're always robustly swimming around in your circulation, ready to swarm and surround any trigger that aims to re-activate your pain and your old destructive patterns.

If you still find yourself being thrown into survival mode dysfunctionally – that is, for a reason that clearly doesn't impact your survival in the least – your first job is to get out of survival mode so you can transition back to homeostasis. You can repeat to yourself this truth: "My survival is not at risk. I'm safe." Becoming aware of and trying to reverse survival-mode-induced changes in the body also acts as a neural antibody that can release you from an addiction alter. So relax your shoulders, unclench your jaws, take several slow, deep breaths. Your conscious mind is speaking to your unconscious mind – because if your unconscious mind really knew, really *got*, that your survival is not at all at risk, it would loosen its grip and let you come back into homeostasis.

Interventions are so useful in fighting addiction in part because, if you let them, they will provide you with very powerful and permanent neural antibodies. The main challenge, particularly with painful life interventions, is not to develop a *new* addiction to the intervention. The strongest addictions probably require several neural antibodies to neutralize them, just as the most virulent strains of bacteria and viruses need to be attacked by the immune system on several fronts. But once your neural antibodies are successfully mobilized to overcome a trigger for any of your addictions, your mind and body will never forget. The whole process will be very strongly reinforced, and then eventually those neural antibodies, when needed, can be mobilized effortlessly and almost automatically.

You and your neural antibodies need to be a team. You're the one who creates your neural antibodies, although all of them *want* to live and, in a real sense, already exist inside you. Once they've been created, you can help them by not forgetting about them – you feed them and keep them strong by reinforcing them, implementing them whenever they can help you see the truth. If you do this, they will be the best, most loving friends you could possibly imagine. If you love and nurture them, your neural antibodies will deliver you from addiction.

Your neural antibodies are your fairy godmothers, your guardian angels. But understand that they are a manifestation of the True Self– of *your* True Self. Do whatever you can to nourish them. Visualize them, give them names, voices, personalities, genders, write down what each one says, what they mean, and where they come from. Do whatever you have to do to make them come alive, to give them life. But let your neural antibodies live. If you let them live, if you nurture them, they will always be there for you. Your neural antibodies come from the True Self, and they will always lead you back to the True Self.

CHAPTER 13

PLAY, DREAMING, AND SELF-DISCOVERY

When animals, particularly mammals, are not in survival mode, when their survival isn't threatened and they don't feel like sleeping, they very often want to play. Animals have relatively limited forms of play, like running, jumping, chasing, or being playfully rough-and-tumble. During our long evolution, we human beings have taken the same primal play instinct that drives animal play and expanded it into every conceivable realm. All humor and verbal banter are forms of play. Sports, art, literature, and music also arise, at least in large part, from this same ancient biological drive to play.

Play probably serves many purposes. During play, animals and people can practice, in a relatively "safe" way, muscle movements that are necessary for fending off attackers or rivals and for finding food and mates. More complex types of play probably also evolved because they allow animals and humans to explore their social environment and the different "roles" that are occupied in that environment. A young girl, for example, gets more insight into the life and responsibilities of a mother when she plays the role of "mother" with her doll. Similarly, during play a smaller dog that is generally more submissive in "real" life can experience what it's like to have a more dominant role when it pounces on a bigger dog that is rolling on its back and playfully assuming a more submissive role.

Survival-mode states are the enemy of play. Animals who are hungry, afraid, or in pain simply don't feel playful. Young vervet monkeys in east Africa, for example, won't play in dry years or times of drought when food is scarce. And when rats are exposed even briefly to the scent of a fox, their natural predator, the rats become afraid and may not play for days. When people are physically ill – clearly a state of survival mode – they don't feel very playful either, and pediatricians, for example, know that when sick children start to laugh and joke again, it's a very favorable sign that the children are getting healthier.

Pure play is a state of flow where we're fully engaged in the present moment, and nothing else exists for us aside from that continuous unfolding moment. Play also generates enormous supplies of healthy, biochemical payoffs. To be healthy, we *need* to play. Hunter-gatherers are very often immersed in playful activities, at least when they're not enduring a drought, food shortage, or other dangerous circumstance. They frequently dance and sing and tell entertaining, funny stories. And they so freely mix work and play that they don't seem to view hunting or gathering as "work" or drudgery at all. Their lives aren't always easy, but it seems safe to say that the average hunter-gatherer spends far more time in pure play mode than the average modern person.

Addiction corrupts play in several different ways. Most importantly, addiction creates a false state of survival mode that will biologically mute the drive to play. If you're chronically anxious because you're addicted to anxiety, for example, you won't feel very playful. You'll often seem to others to be over-serious, not necessarily much fun, and not very prone to good-humored banter. If you're always angry or in emotional or physical pain, you probably also won't feel like playing much. And if you *are* playful, it will often be a little forced, mainly for appearances. If you have to really *try* to be playful, you'll at best be a little split about the experience. And biochemically, you won't be getting nearly as much endorphin from play as people who give themselves over completely to the state of flow when they play. This sets up another self-reinforcing addictive loop: the less you play, the fewer healthy payoffs you get from play; and the fewer healthy payoffs you get from play, the more you'll be driven towards addictive payoffs, which will create survival-mode states that will in turn make you less playful.

Addiction also often turns whatever play we do end up engaging in into a "less than" compensation. Modern culture so relentlessly drives most of us into varying degrees of "less than" that it creates an enormous compensatory drive for us to try to somehow be "more than." This is partly what creates the remarkable obsession with winning found in most modern cultures. Many anthropologists have reported that games and play in hunter-gatherer cultures are largely non-competitive – and on the occasions when hunter-gatherers *are* competitive, their competition is usually fairly discreet. It's usually considered poor taste for any member of a hunter-gatherer band to hold himself or herself higher than other people in the band. Hunter-gatherers do notice, of course, whatever exceptional talents, skills, and physical attributes different band members may possess. But it's generally considered very poor manners to point these talents and attributes out. By nearly all accounts, hunter-gatherer cultures go to great lengths to "level" all the members of the band so that no one feels excessively "more than" or "less than." Hunter-gatherers seem to be acutely aware that strong feelings of "less than" and "more than" can become dangerous threats to the harmony and stability of the groups that they rely on for their survival.

In modern life, on the other hand, many people go to great lengths to put people down, to place themselves above others. And nothing makes us feel so clearly "more than" than being the victors in a game with clearly defined winners and losers – where there's no ambiguity and not much room for interpretation about who's "more than" and who's "less than." When you win, you win.

The problem is that the obsession with winning very often drains play of its joy. In modern culture, even art forms like music and dance that should rightfully have nothing to do with competition, are made into contests and "battles" with winners and losers. If you're only supposed to feel good when you win, and if, as is typically the case in any broad competition, there are more losers than winners, then most people will end up not necessarily feeling so well after a competition. This may even be true if the "competition" concerns a higher art form that is inherently non-competitive.

Winning at games does improve status, and, in an evolutionary sense, there's a substantial benefit to that. But many people are obsessed with winning at games, like video games or tiddlywinks, that will very rarely increase their status in any significant way. That's when things really become dysfunctional. The *need* to win and not be "less than" introduces a survival-mode state into play that is profoundly corrupting.

Since the addiction persona thinks your survival is always at risk, it will interpret a carefree state of flow as being somehow dangerous. The addiction persona, as a manifestation of the addictive drive, will therefore be directly "threatened" by a pure state of play. The addiction persona will often try to pull you out of flow, into an alert, fearful state, or into an apparently urgent "more than" compensation for feelings of "less than." Addiction often corrupts flow states by, for example, compulsively generating obsessive, distracting thoughts that trigger states of survival mode.

People who have tried to meditate, but struggle to do so, face the same dynamic. The addiction persona will often intrude on the homeostatic intention to meditate because the pure state of "being" and tranquility that meditation can provide can seem like a survival risk: if you're completely at peace then you won't be alert or hyper-alert to the many dangers the addiction persona knows are lurking somewhere. The addiction persona becomes so used to steering the ship that when it loses control to the homeostatic drive, it panics and wants urgently to steer again.

Although states of play uncorrupted by addiction can sometimes appear to be relatively serious, they always have a lightness about them, a sense of joy and fun. When you're truly playing, you're intensely alive, throwing all of yourself into it, with little thought about what else you might be doing. This pure state of flow unadulterated by addiction is the key element in any great athletic, dramatic, or musical performance. When you're in a state of flow, you are completely *you*. You're connected to and absorbed in something that's profoundly important and satisfying to you. Addiction often creates an imitation of flow, but true states of flow, unlike addictive states, never have a hangover, they never lead to a swing back of the survival-mode pendulum like addictive states do.

Any kind of judgment will corrupt the state of flow. As soon as there's judgment, the joyful, flowing river of play will quickly become a motionless column of ice. As soon as there's judgment, there's no flow. Thinking about someone laughing at or diminishing what you're doing, for instance, especially when you're doing it earnestly and lovingly, can instantly interrupt your state of flow and take you out of the present moment and homeostasis.

But much of the time, that judgment is actually created by *you*. It's often something *you're* thinking, some way that you're judging *yourself*, and not necessarily anything that someone else is thinking. And even if people *are* judging you, those judgments almost always arise out of their own feelings of "less than" and rarely represent anything remotely approaching a survival risk for you. The fear of judgment breeds survival-mode states that are typically completely illusory.

The play instinct can also be manipulated and distorted by addiction in a more subtle way. All addiction alters can be seen, at least at one level, as unconscious manipulations of the play instinct. The alters, when we get triggered into them, are dysfunctional "roles" that we play, and when we play any "role" in our lives, we're using the spirit and instinct of play dysfunctionally. Playing a role feeds addiction because it always involves a disconnection between your core self and the specific impression you're trying to make on other people with the alter, or "character," that you've created. It's one thing if such a role comes from a spirit of play, like a child playing mother to her doll. But it's a very different thing when that role is who you really think you are, or who you convince yourself that you need to be to get what you want, or just to "survive."

If, for example, your parents reinforced what a sweet girl you were as a child, and chastised you, made you feel ashamed or "less than" if you were not "sweet," then you probably grew up thinking that you needed to be "sweet" to be okay, to get what you wanted, to be accepted and loved. It wasn't enough to just be who you were – you needed to be extra sweet all the time, even when you didn't feel so well emotionally or physically. But no one is "sweet" a hundred percent of the time. And so that creates a disconnection within you.

Playing a "role" in your life is to be overly invested in how other people perceive you. And what if they don't respond to you in the way that you would like them to? Then you'll often crash into desperate, unsettled feelings of "less than." And even when you do get the response you want when you play your role, the experience will still be disconnecting because then you'll feel that people aren't responding to the authentic you. At some level, you yourself will probably even begin to believe that you somehow *are* the role that you play, and so you will become even further disconnected both from other people and from your own core self. When you're acting out of addiction, it's always like that – you're going to lose either way.

If you're in a bad mood and aren't acting so sweet, you may feel ashamed or "less than," because you've violated the role you think you need to play to be "enough," to be okay. And if you do always behave sweetly, you'll inevitably be submerging less-than-sweet thoughts and impulses, and that will create a non-homeostatic, addiction-propelling disconnection within you. The only homeostatic solution is for you to be *you* – to be connected to your core self rather than to some abstract, imaginary, play-like role that you've been unconsciously saddled with. Being "sweet" has become a fragmented, split-off symbol of your self. You may often act sweetly, but when you do so, it should be authentic, it should come from *you*.

If we're going to beat addiction, we need to play in healthy, and not dysfunctional, ways. Among other things, play can help us to recover the full capacity to *feel*, which is a critical element in overcoming addiction. Activities like dance or yoga, where the body can become an active vehicle for feeling, can be especially beneficial. Frequent dancing is a universal aspect of hunter-gatherer cultures. In dance, the body can, in effect, be "danced" by the music and the rhythm – there can be a letting go of the obsessive need of the mind to control the body out of exaggerated safety concerns. Physical movement can also interrupt addictive cycles by using the dopamine build-up in the brain not to crave or obsess, but to actually *move*, to take action, to play.

The biological drive that compels us to play probably arises from many of the same circuits in the brain that lead us to dream while we sleep. Numerous similarities exist between play states and dreaming states. Dopamine, for example, is an important neurochemical not only for play and addiction, but also for dreaming. Although many researchers have argued that dreams serve no useful or functional biological purpose, this seems extremely unlikely. Like almost everything else about us at a basic biological level, dreams probably evolved to help us survive, reproduce, and maintain states of homeostasis.

Dreams can be extraordinarily complex, and often appear to have several layers of purpose or meaning. But, in a simple sense, a dream may serve the homeostatic drive by highlighting some present or future danger that the dreamer is either not fully conscious of or is not taking the appropriate action to combat or prepare for. When a hunter-gatherer is facing a true survival risk, his or her dreams will presumably be doing all they can to help devise the most functional response to those risks during waking life.

But while the great majority of hunter-gatherer dreams are likely to be functional, or at least not harmful, in modern life many dreams appear to be addiction dreams. That is, just as we often think of something painful or distressing in waking life to get a dysfunctional payoff, particular dreams often create distressing thoughts or feelings within us that don't seem to serve any purpose aside from providing a drug payoff. Whatever emotional addictions you have in waking life will almost certainly arise in some or most of your dreams as well. If you have an addiction to anxiety, for example, you'll also tend to have a lot of anxiety dreams – dreams that create feelings of anxiety for no apparently functional or illuminating purpose.

Dreams are corrupted by addiction when part of the unconscious mind is tricked into thinking that survival is at risk when it is not. In that case dreams, like so much else in modern life, will simply become dysfunctional. Nightmares, for example, or very unpleasant dreams that could qualify as nightmares, evolved to help us either process or foresee survival-related traumas. But in modern life, the great majority of nightmares, and nearly all repetitive nightmares, are probably driven, either directly or indirectly, by addiction. When we wake up feeling depressed or pained, the reason is often that we've had a particularly nasty addiction dream. After you wake up from an intense anxiety dream, for instance, you may feel at least a little more anxious than usual for the rest of the day.

As you overcome your addictions, one by one, you'll generally find that your dreams will become far more pleasant. Just as we tend to be more playful in waking life if we perceive our circumstances to be relatively safe, if we don't feel that our survival is threatened during waking life, our *dreams* will also tend to be more like play states. As you overcome more and more of your addictions, your dreams, if you pay attention to them, will become more interesting and provocative, even funny, and will often provide deep insights into your own circumstances. In short, when we're consistently in survival mode during waking life, our dreams will often be more like nightmares; but when we're *not* typically in survival mode during waking life, our dreams will often be more like play.

With less addiction, your dreams will serve the homeostatic drive in the narrow sense of minimizing your pain and distress, but also in the broad sense of helping you to grow emotionally, intellectually, and spiritually. Just as looking at various issues from different viewpoints can broaden and deepen our intellectual appreciation of the world, dreams and play states create scenarios that allow us to look at our own experiences from a slightly different angle, which can facilitate personal growth.

Dream researchers like Kelly Bulkeley have written extensively about the enormous emotional and spiritual impact of expansive, "big" dreams that people from every known culture have been found to experience. Dreams are like nightly works of art that can have profound and mysterious effects on us. Hundreds, perhaps thousands, of dreams have inspired lasting works of art or important scientific discoveries. Without addiction, many of us would be similarly inspired, in countless and complicated ways, by our own dreams. The more your dreams can be unsullied by addiction, the more access you will have to dreams that will provide you with both practical and spiritual illumination.

When you begin to have fewer addiction dreams, your dreams will start working for you in many ways. They may also help you to directly *overcome* addiction. The pioneering dream researcher William Dement, for example, who coined the term "REM sleep" – the sleep phase during which dreaming predominantly occurs – had an extraordinarily vivid dream that changed his life and acted, in our terminology, as an intervention. At the time of the dream, Dement was a heavy cigarette smoker. He dreamed that he went for a check-up and his doctor found an inoperable cancer of the lung. During the dream, Dement wrote, "I experienced the incredible anguish of knowing my life was soon to end, that I would never see my children grow up... I will never forget the surprise, joy, and exquisite relief of waking up. I felt I was reborn." After the dream, Dement immediately stopped smoking cigarettes, apparently for good.

When dreams arise from the functional, homeostatic drive, they can also help you overcome a variety of emotional addictions. If you're angry at someone and have become addicted to that anger, for example, you may have a dream that shows you how much pain this particular person is in. In waking life, it may be hard for you to let go of your anger towards the person, but the dream may cut through that anger by highlighting the pain that almost always lies beneath hurtful behavior. This kind of dream, just like a life intervention during waking life, is trying hard to shift you back into homeostasis by getting you to see and process something that part of you doesn't want to see.

Typically, the reason you'll be resistant to really seeing or facing particular truths is that if you *did* see those truths clearly and fully, you would have to give up an addiction and overcome some false state of survival mode that the addiction is perpetuating. When you have such dreams, and pay attention to them, they can initiate a positive, self-reinforcing *homeostatic* loop: the more you work during waking life to overcome your addictions, the fewer addiction dreams you will have, and so the more your dreams can serve their natural function of helping to bring you back into homeostasis. The less addiction you have in your dreams, the more you can avail yourself of the riches that dreams have to offer.

Of course you won't be able to dream as much or be responsive to those dreams if you can't fall asleep in the first place. If you're in survival mode, your mind thinks your survival is at risk, and so it will release copious amounts of stress hormones like adrenaline and cortisol that will put your system on high alert, and will create the illusion that it's a dangerous time to sleep. That's why when you're immersed in any emotional addiction, such as an addiction to anger, worry, or fear, you'll often have a very difficult time getting a good night's sleep.

When we're out of balance, our minds and bodies send us signals that are trying to tell us to do certain things, to make certain decisions that will bring us back into balance. If we haven't been getting enough sleep, our brains and bodies will signal to us that we're tired, and will try to get us to take a nap, or to sleep longer during the night. But instead of responding to these signals by sleeping more, many people in modern life instead drink coffee or stimulant-laden "energy" drinks. Although these drinks will certainly be temporarily energizing, they will also severely disrupt the homeostatic drive.

When your body is trying to get you back into balance by getting you to sleep more, but you instead override its signals and just feed it more caffeine, you're subverting the homeostatic drive. You're not allowing the healthiest and most powerful force in your mind and body to do its work, to operate correctly. Consistently drinking coffee instead of getting more sleep not only creates a coffee addiction, but will also make you more prone to other addictions, such as emotional addictions, since the pattern will make it much more difficult for you to remain in a stable state of homeostasis. When we're getting enough sleep, it's far easier for us to be in homeostasis and far easier for us to overcome our addictions.

As you overcome your addictive patterns, you will reap the benefits of sleeping better, feeling more playful, and having more pleasant dreams. Your dreams and play will also become powerful vehicles for self-discovery. And the more you know and discover about yourself, the less prone you will be to further addiction. It always helps to ask yourself: what do I really want? What's most important to me? When I'm close to death and I look back on my life, what will I want to have accomplished? What kind of person would I like to have been? When you start to feel a truer sense of your own purpose, of your homeostatic drive, and become more fully connected to that purpose and drive, addiction will begin to lose its power over you.

CHAPTER 14

THE NOW/HOMEOSTASIS CONTINUUM

Part of what makes us unique as a species is our powerful ability to mentally "travel" through time by creating images in our minds that represent the past or the future. All other animals, to varying degrees, seem to be far more tied to the present – they can't escape from the present moment by imagining themselves in the past or the future to the same extent that we can. "Mental time travel" is a critical part of human consciousness and an essential element in higher art and creativity. And yet it is also responsible, directly or indirectly, for most of our psychological dysfunctions. All of our emotional addictions, for example, would be far less potent, if not impossible, without our capacity to call up painful images from the past, or to imagine future scenarios that provoke anxiety.

A key concept in Buddhism, as in many other spiritual traditions, is the importance of living in the present moment, of not getting lost in thoughts about the past and the future. But given that mental time travel is so critical to being human, it's important to have a sense of when it is and is not appropriate or healthy to think about the past or the future. The model described in this book greatly clarifies this issue. When thoughts about the future or the past are being engaged in repetitively and compulsively, when memories of the past or projections into the future create clear states of survival mode that drive a stress response, the pattern is almost certainly dysfunctional. But if thoughts about the past and the future act as part of a creative process or a form of play, or are serving some other functional purpose, they are more likely to be a true expression of being fully alive.

While there has been a great deal of attention paid to living in the "present moment," or in the "Now," the pure experience of the "Now" probably evolved to allow us to best respond to survival emergencies, or to situations that were clear threats to our survival and

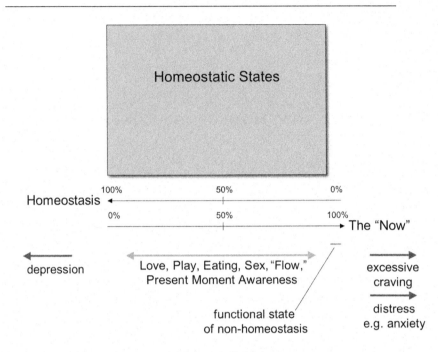

Figure 7: The Now/Homeostasis continuum. Any point along the continuum represents a functional state. A pure (100%) state of the "Now" is the only functional state of survival-mode, or non-homeostasis. A pure (100%) state of homeostasis would be, for example, a state of deep meditation. All states along the continuum represent different types of homeostasis, with different levels, or percentages, of "pure" homeostasis, mixed in with different levels, or percentages, of the "Now." Any point outside of this continuum represents a dysfunctional survival-mode state driven by addiction.

reproduction. In a pure state of the Now, colors are more vibrant, time slows down, the senses are intensely alert. We can imagine our hunter-gatherer ancestors in a state of the Now walking through a forest or savannah full of dangerous predators. In such a circumstance, being in the Now would be the most functional state.

But with no apparent survival threats around, a pure state of the Now would be inappropriate. Why not relax a bit? Why not move towards homeostasis? This is what all other animals do. A domestic cat, for example, simulates a state of the Now when it's stalking a bird or a mouse – if the cat were in the wild, successful hunting would be critical for its survival, and the more alert its senses, the better. But when survival is not directly at risk, cats, like all other animals, shift towards a calm, relaxed, peaceful state of homeostasis. Similarly, when hunter-gatherers are out of danger, when they've just eaten and are sitting with the rest of the band around the fires that are protective against predators, they are unlikely to be in a pure state of the Now. They are much more likely to be in a state closer to homeostasis.

It's probably not appropriate, functional, or healthy to be in a pure state of the Now unless survival is directly at risk. A pure state of the Now – as we're defining it here – can be thought of as the only completely functional state of non-homeostasis, or survival mode. Therefore trying too hard to be in the Now can potentially perpetuate non-homeostasis. When people are always seeking to live in the Now, they may not necessarily end up being very homeostatic or peaceful, and may instead unwittingly move towards a more hyper-alert, emergency state. On the other hand, many people may not want to be in a "pure" state of homeostasis, such as deep meditation, for too much of their lives either.

It's therefore useful to imagine a continuum that lies between a pure state of homeostasis and a pure state of the Now (Figure 7). A pure, 100% state of the Now is only appropriate for a survival-related circumstance. But anywhere else along the continuum between a pure state of the Now and a pure state of homeostasis would be optimal and functional for various life circumstances, and would potentially represent healthy, vital states of flow. When our survival is not directly at risk – which is very often the case in modern life – we can *choose* which position along the continuum feels best given our current circumstances and state of mind. We may choose to be more relaxed and calm, perhaps even to meditate, which will be closer to pure homeostasis; or we may choose to be boisterous and exuberant, and perhaps physically active or playful, which would take us closer to a pure state of the Now. Within this continuum, therefore, homeostasis and the Now would be blended to various degrees. Sometimes there would be a dominant feeling of the Now, and at other times there would be a dominant feeling of homeostasis.

Anywhere outside of this continuum, however, can be thought of as a dysfunctional state. If we go beyond a feeling of being in the Now, we may become hyper-active, hyper-sexual, or overly anxious. If we're overly craving food, sex, or other kinds of artificial "excite-ment," we'll be thrown out of a flow state into a state of survival mode, a state of *need*. If we move too far in the other direction, beyond a state of being relaxed and peaceful, we may feel lethargic and depressed, which represents another type of survival mode. If we're completely healthy and functional, even if we're in extreme physical or emotional pain, we would never go further than being in the Now with that pain. In the Now we would be fully *experiencing* the pain, but would not become *attached* to it – we wouldn't be *using* the pain, prolonging it or exaggerating it or somehow making it worse than it is just to get an enhanced biochemical payoff from it.

When you're deep in a non-homeostatic survival-mode state, such as a state of severe emotional pain, it's very difficult, in practice, to shift directly back into homeostasis. The easiest way to transition back, and often the only way, is to first come back into a pure state of present moment awareness that most closely approximates how we're defining the Now. After you're in the Now, you can more easily find your way back to homeostasis. This is probably how we evolved biologically: when we're in a survival-related situation, our brains want to bring us into the Now, because that's the most functional way to deal with a survival threat. Then when the threat passes, we can shift back into homeostasis.

Similarly, if we're in survival mode for a *dysfunctional* reason – that is, because of addiction – coming into the Now is usually the best way to transition back to homeostasis. One powerful way of coming into the Now after being in survival mode is to try to more fully engage your senses: observe what's around you, listen to the sounds in your environment, connect to your sense of touch. Using your senses can interrupt dysfunctional, addictive thought patterns to bring you back into the present moment and ultimately into homeostasis.

Addictive patterns are almost always distorted, dysfunctional attempts to bring us back into the Now. The manic, high-energy phase of bipolar disorder, for example, which often involves hyper-sexuality or uncontrollable spending of money, can be seen in large part as a dysfunctional attempt to feel, to be in the Now, to be *alive*. Similarly, "cutters" cut themselves partly so they can *feel*, and that intense feeling of a fresh cut, a fresh injury, will, at least at some level, also bring them into the "Now." But it's a dysfunctional strategy – first because it's based on pain, on getting a payoff from pain and injury; and, second, because it generates shame and other negative emotions that will make it even more difficult to be in a healthy, functional state of homeostasis.

Hunter-gatherers have a relatively easy time staying alert to the present moment, largely because they are constantly immersed in the natural world, which is always enthralling. Being surrounded by nature tends to keep most of us in the present moment and out of obsessive thought patterns. For a hunter-gatherer in particular, obsessive thinking at the expense of present moment awareness is also potentially life-threatening. If a hunter-gatherer becomes too immersed in addictive mental chatter and is not sufficiently careful or alert, he or she may not, for instance, notice a slithering poisonous snake that could deliver a fatal bite.

The extent to which someone is "present" can be seen as the extent to which he or she is not receiving a dysfunctional drug payoff in that moment. Being in the "present" then really just means, in this sense, not to be deriving any dysfunctional biochemical payoffs at that moment. You may, for example, be doing imaginative work that involves calling up images of the past or the future – but if those images aren't driven by addiction, if you're not getting an addictive payoff from them, if you're not in a false state of survival mode, then operationally you'll still be somewhere along the Now/Homeostasis continuum.

When we recall an image from the past, that image is "called up" in our minds using the same part of the brain, called the visual cortex, that is utilized to process scenes that we are actually looking at in the present moment. Studies have shown that when people are visualizing images in their minds called up from the past, they literally don't see what's in front of them as well as they normally would. This is because so much of the activity and space in the visual cortex is already being used to "view," in the mind's eye, the visual image that is displayed in one's imagination. Thus visual images are "viewed" at the expense, to varying degrees, of the real images and scenes that are in front of our eyes. When we become excessively absorbed in visual images from the past, therefore, we quite literally don't *see* as well in the present, and aren't as available to fully experience the present moment. If recalling a particular image from the past is serving some functional or creative purpose, there's nothing necessarily unhealthy about the recollection or the image. But if the image is only being recalled or imagined to stimulate unnecessary anger, self-pity, or regret, for example, then it's being driven by addiction. In this case, addiction would be directly intruding on our full experience of being alive and of actually *seeing* our environment.

In the spiritual and enlightenment literature, particularly in Buddhism, there is much discussion about being fully "awake." The Buddha was the "awakened one," someone who had attained full spiritual enlightenment. People who are not enlightened or awakened are, to varying degrees, still "asleep," living in a cloud of illusion. The model we have presented in this book suggests a clear biochemical underpinning for this notion. That is, people who live their lives within the Now/Homeostasis continuum, like the Buddha was reputed to have done after his awakening, would be considered enlightened. Other people – the vast majority, at minimum, of people who are alive today – spend significant portions, if not almost all, of their time living outside of that continuum.

Whenever people spend time outside of the Now/Homeostasis continuum, they will be receiving dysfunctional payoffs from artificial survival-mode states. They may receive "stimulants" from, for example, excessive craving for food or sex, or from unnecessary states of anxiety or fear. And they may receive "depressants" from painful thoughts about the past, or from feelings of self-pity or hopelessness.

When people are in these dysfunctional, unnecessary, non-homeostatic states of survival mode, they are quite literally being "drugged." Being outside of the Now/Homeostasis continuum is very much like being under the influence of a narcotic. People who are under the influence of substantial amounts of alcohol or addictive drugs are never quite "there," they are partly unconscious, and are only using a small portion of the potential range of their consciousness. Similarly, people who often operate outside of the Now/Homeostasis continuum, even if they never use addictive drugs or alcohol, are using their emotions and obsessive thought patterns to supply the direct *equivalent* of such drugs. Although they may be formally "conscious," they are also largely "asleep," not fully awake to the present moment. They are certainly not in a state of "flow" or homeostasis.

Emotional addicts are therefore being "drugged" by their own stress hormones, and thus are not fully "awake." Obsessive, addictive mental chatter always makes people more narcissistic, more "in their own worlds." That chatter makes it much more difficult to really listen to other people, for example, to really take in other people and try to connect with them. Emotional addicts may not always be quite as "zoned-out" as substance abusers or alcoholics, but they will not be in a state of flow, and will not be fully alive.

Thus if you aspire to be "awakened" or enlightened, like the Buddha, Jesus, or other great spiritual teachers were reputed to have been, you would need to overcome the addictions that keep you, to varying degrees, in a "drugged" state. If you were living exclusively within the Now/Homeostasis continuum, and only transitioned into a pure state of the Now during true survival emergencies, you would be fully awake. You would be living purely out of the homeostatic drive and the True Self.

CHAPTER 15

HIGHER LEVELS OF HOMEOSTASIS

When our survival is truly at risk, the addiction persona becomes irrelevant in most cases, because it will be telling us the same message as the rest of the brain: if you don't do something fast, you really *are* going to die. But even when life is just about surviving, the homeostatic drive and the True Self are still your best guides. The True Self does it all: it helps you reach the highest levels of spiritual fulfillment, and it helps you to survive when your life is truly in peril.

Homeostasis at its first and most basic level strives simply to keep nutrients, minerals, and other biomolecules in balance within all the cells of our brains and bodies. The second level of homeostasis involves complex emotional states that motivate us to make specific decisions, or perform specific actions, that will enhance our survival prospects. At this second level the homeostatic drive includes a force that seeks to keep both our cells and our *emotions* in an appropriate balance.

The first two levels of homeostasis are mostly about survival. All other animals also operate according to these basic principles. But there is a third level of homeostasis that is clearly vastly more developed in humans than in other animals, and may well be exclusive to humans. This third level involves personal, artistic, intellectual, and spiritual fulfillment. Although such higher "needs," when fulfilled, will also often improve status – which in a biological sense, will enhance survival prospects – there's also an aspect to this level that can transcend any survival or reproductive concerns. The desire to be an artist, for instance, may become a higher need, just as water and food are more basic needs. If true painters don't paint, if they don't express through painting what they somehow need to express, something akin to hunger will keep tugging at them. They will generally find it far easier to be in homeostasis when they paint than when they don't paint.

This third level of homeostasis concerns the True Self at its highest levels. Artists, for example, are driven by some guiding force within them that indicates which direction they should follow to fulfill their potential as artists. This guiding force can only be the drive to homeostasis. When mere survival becomes less challenging, or when personal survival concerns can somehow be transcended, relationships with other people also begin to involve this third level. Being in a friendship or romantic relationship largely out of status concerns is a remnant of our evolutionary heritage as hunter-gatherers, when survival was always at issue, and when developing relationships with high-status people notably increased one's chances of survival and reproduction.

In modern life, people who are not driven repeatedly and falsely into survival mode due to their addictive patterns are more likely to embrace the higher aspects of the third level of homeostasis. Because feelings of "less than" ultimately drive nearly all addictive patterns, if you do not often experience these feelings, if you are not prone to a "less than" addiction, you're much less likely to enter into a relationship purely or largely because of status concerns or addiction-driven control dramas. The less addiction you have in your life, therefore, the more balanced, content, and peaceful you will be, and the more you will be influenced by the highest, most transcendent level of the homeostatic drive. Like all levels of the homeostatic drive, this highest level is expressed through the True Self.

There's a long and somewhat complicated tradition in Christianity called Gnosticism that is also specifically concerned with the True Self. The Gnostics believe that the True Self is the portal to all spiritual and religious experience, and that achieving self-knowledge – specifically knowledge of the True Self – is tantamount to salvation. Carl Jung, who embraced the main tenets of Gnosticism, said that the True Self is the "God-image" within the human psyche. While we are not capable of knowing conclusively at this point whether or not there is a "God," Jung said, there is clearly a God-*image* within the psyche of every man and woman that responds intensely to religious images and symbols. This God-image, Jung and the Gnostics believed, is the True Self, our authentic or higher selves. Anyone who knows the True Self, therefore, will, in effect, know God.

Jung believed that while Christ was a true prophet, a deeply enlightened spiritual teacher of genius, Christ also became a symbol of the higher self, a symbol of what it's like to live purely out of the True Self. Eastern religions such as Buddhism explicitly suggest that God is not external to man, but rather internal to man. God is *within* man. The Buddha, for example, said that if he was a "God," then so too was every other human being. The Buddha portrayed himself as just an ordinary man who happened to awaken to the secret of spiritual enlightenment, and he insisted that his disciples should not worship him as a God. According to both Buddhism and to a Gnostic interpretation of Christianity, in other words, all human beings have God within them.

Many scholars, such as Elaine Pagels, a Professor of Religion at Princeton University, have argued that the core teachings of Jesus are very similar to the teachings of the Buddha, and that the teachings of Jesus were grossly distorted and misinterpreted both by his disciples and by the early Christian Church. Jung argued that Jesus made desperate attempts to teach his disciples *not* to imitate him. Jesus implored the disciples to live their *own* lives – that is, to live out of their own True Selves. Only *then* would they be like Jesus, and only then would they themselves, in effect, be Gods. But the disciples did not understand what Jesus meant, Jung said, and they took Jesus himself to be God. The true message of Christ, Jung and the Gnostics suggested, is that we all have to live our *own* lives, to find our *own* True Self, and only *that* will lead us to a true experience of God. Jesus, in this view, is not so much an external manifestation of God, but rather a messenger of the True Self.

Many aspects of the New Testament hint at this interpretation of Christianity. Jung and the Gnostics suggested, for example, that when Jesus said, "The Kingdom of God is within you," he was referring directly to the True Self that is found within all of us. Many Christians have interpreted Jesus's famous proclamation, "I am the way, the truth, and the life: no man cometh unto the Father, but by me" as meaning that the only path to God, or the "Father," is through the practice of traditional Christianity, through worship of Christ. But Carl Jung suggested that this statement actually refers to the *True Self*. Christ is a symbol of the True Self, and so the deeper meaning of this statement is that no one finds God except through the *True Self*.

According to the model presented in this book, a critical part of self-knowledge and knowledge of the True Self is the awareness of one's addictive patterns, and anyone who overcomes his or her addictive patterns will be living purely out of the True Self. The model therefore, in effect, connects the concept of homeostasis, or the drive to homeostasis, which is perhaps the central principle in biology, with the Gnostic idea of the True Self. If you let the homeostatic drive guide you, we've argued, then you will be guided by, or will be living out of, the True Self. So if the True Self does indeed represent the "God-image" within us, if the True Self is the manifestation of God within all of us, then if we commit to the homeostatic drive, and thus commit to the True Self, we will, in effect, be doing "God's will." To commit to homeostasis is therefore to do God's will. Indeed the drive to homeostasis within all of us, and perhaps within all living things, may not just be a *manifestation* of God. The homeostatic drive may itself *be* what many people typically think of as "God": the powerful, invisible, beneficent force that leads us towards peace and tranquility – the gravitational pull that seeks harmony for all things, that binds all things together.

Since addiction is what keeps us apart from the True Self, addiction would then be what keeps us, in effect, apart from God. People who have addictions are certainly not intrinsically evil, or else all of us would be intrinsically evil. But when people talk about the force of evil, about the devil, about Satan, they are, in this view, referring to addiction and the addictive drive.

When we operate out of the addictive, non-homeostatic drive, we allow the dysfunctional part of ourselves to pull us out of balance unnecessarily, into pain or distress. But when we operate out of this same addictive drive, we do the very same thing to *other people* – that is, we unconsciously try to pull *them* out of homeostasis as well. Just as substance abusers have "partying buddies," and alcoholics are always seeking drinking companions, emotional addicts want and need other emotional addicts to "party" with, to be out of balance with. In the most serious relationship dramas, for instance, both people continually drive each other into out-of-balance, survival-mode states like anger, fear, anxiety, guilt, "less than," and self-pity. Non-homeostasis thus not only begets further non-homeostasis within ourselves, but also in the people with whom we interact.

At the simplest level, a person can be passively "infected" by, for example, another person's anger and anxiety. If you're anxious, simply by virtue of you interacting with other people, of you being in their vicinity, there's a greater chance that your anxiety will cause *them* to become anxious also. Non-homeostasis can breed more non-homeostasis, fear and anger can breed more fear and anger. At the most severe level, people may derive substantial unconscious payoffs from directly causing another person pain, or by pointedly trying to make another person feel "less than."

This is why we need, above all, to commit to our *own* homeostasis first. If we ourselves are consistently in non-homeostasis, we will almost always be doing so out of addiction. And if we're operating out of addiction, we will almost inescapably, if unconsciously, be trying to pull other people into non-homeostasis with us, thus causing *them* unnecessary pain and distress. If we're operating out of addiction, even when we convince ourselves that we're just trying to help other people, we'll very likely end up hurting them.

But, on the other hand, if we're committing to *homeostasis*, and operating out of the *homeostatic* drive, we'll want other people to be in *homeostasis* with us. When we feel at peace, when we feel confident, secure, alive, and unthreatened, we want the best for everyone, we wish everyone could feel as good as we do. It's only when we're *out* of balance, when we're pained or distressed, that we can consciously or unconsciously wish other people ill. When we're committed to homeostasis, just as we don't pull *ourselves* out of balance, we don't feel compelled, consciously or unconsciously, to pull other people out of balance either.

Furthermore, if we truly commit to homeostasis within ourselves, we have to find some way of coming into balance with our environment, and especially with other people in our environment. Perhaps the most homeostatic solution regarding one particular person is to become romantically involved with or married to them, and the homeostatic solution regarding another particular person is to see them as seldom as possible. Maybe it's homeostatic to have some fairly severe boundaries on a particular relationship, or even to make sure particular people are put into prison – in some cases, maybe *that's* the boundary that's needed! But if you're going to be fully functional, living authentically out of the homeostatic drive, you have to figure out the best way to come into balance with other people, whatever form your relationship with them will take. As each person in the world begins to interact in this way in all of his or her relationships, it will withdraw dysfunction from those relationships. The more homeostatic the people around us are, the more harmonious it will be for us. The simple commitment to homeostasis within ourselves therefore creates a driving force that will tend to also drive our environment toward homeostasis.

The only real sensor we have for homeostasis is within *ourselves*. Even though it may at first sound selfish, we have to commit above all to our own homeostasis, or we will, paradoxically, end up being *more* selfish, being worse human beings. Because if we don't pay attention to our own homeostatic sensor, addiction will begin to drive us, and soon we'll be unconsciously driving other people towards addiction as well. So if we want to be the best people we can possibly be, if we want to live out of the True Self, if we want to do God's will, we have to commit to our own homeostasis *first*. This general dynamic appears to be inescapable.

The drive to homeostasis therefore fulfills one of the ultimate goals of all the great spiritual and religious traditions: peace, or homeostasis, for all people, and indeed for all things. Being unnecessarily unkind or deceitful towards others will, for many reasons, be non-homeostatic for *you* – partly because a portion of your self will feel, although perhaps unconsciously, shame or guilt about your actions, and partly because being unkind or deceitful will make it far more difficult for you to truly *connect* with other people. And it always feels infinitely better to connect with other people than to throw them out of balance. The homeostatic drive thus supports the Golden Rule: that you should do unto others as you would have them do unto you.

Since anyone who becomes caught in the non-homeostatic drive will inescapably cause himself or herself a great deal of pain, once people become conscious of how the addictive drive operates, the only reason they would *not* seek to overcome their addictions is that they have consciously chosen to give themselves more pain. And that makes no sense at all – very few people, if any, would *consciously* choose to have more pain once they know how addictive dynamics operate. Once people see and experience the peace and transcendent bliss of living out of the True Self, why would they ever choose pain?

This book has provided a path that can be followed to overcome any addiction. The less any addictive pattern is activated, the weaker it will become. And for every addictive pattern that you weaken, for every addiction that you overcome, the closer you will be to the True Self. Knowing what you know now, why would you *not* want to commit to homeostasis and the True Self? Knowing that addiction is likely responsible for all of your chronic emotional pain, and probably, directly or indirectly, for most of your chronic physical pain as well, why would you not seek to overcome all of your addictions?

CONCLUSION

If you can appreciate the full breadth and glory of homeostasis, and how addiction creates a force that directly opposes homeostasis, you'll have grasped the core message in this book. But remember that addiction can be hiding almost anywhere in the psyche. If the whole of you isn't committed to being in a homeostatic state of flow or peace whenever possible, then at least part of you is still under the sway of your addiction alters. If the whole of you doesn't want your emotional and physical pain to be healed, then part of you still wants to use that pain as a drug.

Although addiction always creates or perpetuates *unnecessary* pain, overcoming addiction and growing as a person are usually also not without some pain. We may have to confront pain that we haven't yet sufficiently dealt with, or face the painful loss of part of our previous life as our emotional and spiritual growth advance us forward to a new way of living. But this kind of pain is nothing to be afraid of. As long as you don't get addicted to the pain, as long as you know that the pain must be confronted for you to be whole again, you can always pass through it and come back into balance.

The beauty of how we're built as biological systems is that we have a built-in sensor for all types of emotional and physical balance. That sensor is the feeling of homeostasis. When you're in homeostasis, in flow, there's no "buzz" in the mind, no stress, no neurotic tension. Once you recognize what it truly feels like to be in homeostasis, and how infinitely more pleasant homeostasis feels than being in survival mode, you'll become connected to the drive that will guide you for the rest of your life. If you're truly in homeostasis, then you must be doing the right thing, or at least you must be awfully close. If you're in homeostasis at the deepest level, if you feel that sense of bliss and transcendence that homeostasis will always give rise to, then you *know* you're doing the right thing – you know you're aligning with the deepest and truest part of yourself.

Only addiction stands between you and the drive that can always bring you back into balance. Natural selection could not possibly have foreseen how modern, post-agricultural environments would make human beings so acutely prone to addiction. And it isn't clear how natural selection could possibly have modified our brains to make us less susceptible to addiction within those environments. There was simply no easy way to change the basic biochemistry of the brain at that deep a level, and there still isn't. The potential confusion between pleasure and pain, between excitement and distress, is too deeply embedded in the brain's basic operating system. Only consciousness of how addiction works and how it can be healed will allow us to truly overcome our addictive patterns.

Although addiction is really just a strange illusion, a trick of the mind, it can corrupt every part of you. Addiction takes your self, your glorious, perfectly-crafted harp, and bludgeons the strings with a hammer. If you've never heard just how beautifully that harp can play, the sound addiction makes can seem like music. But after addiction plays, you always feel worse than you did before it began, and it always leaves blood on the stage. Addiction can hold you in a spell, but it knows only one song: the music of survival, played with a false and destructive urgency.

The truth will unwind and unravel any addiction. When the truth causes you pain, it will be a necessary pain, the pain of confronting how lost you've been, how so much of your life has been lived in a fog. Homeostasis is the call from the True Self that will lead you back home. The pull of homeostasis is the whisper of God's love.

BACKGROUND & ACKNOWLEDGMENTS

The model described in this book developed out of a collaboration between me and Todd Ritchey. Although the book was written entirely by me, many of Todd's phrases, analogies, and stories also found their way into the text, particularly in Chapters 8 – 12.

I first met Todd and his wife Stacy in September, 2004 in a small coffee shop in Redondo Beach, California when they were in the audience while I was performing as a singer-songwriter. I didn't see them again until almost exactly a year later, in September, 2005. I was touring along the west coast as a musician, playing mainly in bars and coffee shops, and drove to Vancouver, British Columbia, where Todd, Stacy, and their children had recently moved. Shortly after I arrived at their house, Todd told me about a meditation he had had the previous week. This meditation supplied a number of the initial ideas for the model.

As Todd described the experience, a series of images came to him for what seemed like only a few seconds during the eighth minute of his meditation. After he came out of his meditative state, he translated those images into several ideas, which mainly concerned addiction and which he hurriedly wrote down. Todd had been doing interventions and counseling for many years, and already had a great deal of experience with and knowledge about addiction. He had also created his own unique method of doing counseling and interventions, often combining spiritual perspectives with the more traditional tools of psychotherapy. Although Todd had little formal education or training, from the first night I met him I sensed he was a true student of human nature and that he had an extraordinary intuition about how people operate. This initial impression has since been repeatedly confirmed.

These were the main ideas that I took away from what Todd told me about this remarkable meditation:

1. People can become addicted to negative emotional states such as anxiety, and to other mental states such as needing to be "right."
2. These addictions work the same way as addictive drugs.
3. Feelings of "less than" drive all addictions.
4. All addictions are linked together in the brain through an associative neural network, which Todd called the "addiction persona." The addiction persona acts almost as a separate personality.
5. All addictions work by hijacking the survival instincts.
6. Addiction is responsible for nearly all chronic emotional and physical pain, and all psychological dysfunction.
7. If people could rid themselves of all of their addictions, they would be living purely out of their authentic selves, which would allow them to connect more deeply to their own experiences of love and creativity.
8. This suggested a new way of doing psychotherapy. Addressing people's addictions would be a direct way to help them overcome their blocks.
9. One powerful way to overcome addiction would be to "mute" the triggers for those addictions.

There weren't many other details from the meditation, but I was immediately intrigued by these ideas, several of which I had never heard before. Todd and I decided at the end of my visit that we would pursue the ideas further and write a book about them. After I left Vancouver, I became increasingly focused on the implications of the ideas. It seemed to me that they suggested a new way of looking at a number of classical issues in psychology, neuroscience, and spirituality.

It took several years of intensive work for many of the core ideas in the model as it currently stands to take shape. These later ideas came mainly from my own work, but were often refined and explored further during conversations with Todd. Some of the ideas discussed in the first several chapters and in Chapter 13 came about within the first year. It wasn't until the beginning of the third year of work that I realized how the concept of homeostasis could serve as the unifying framework for the entire model. Viewing psychological processes through the lens of homeostatic forces was impressed upon me partly by Bud Craig, a neuroscientist at the Barrow Neurological Institute in Phoenix, Arizona, whose papers I read carefully and with whom I had a phone conversation that affected me greatly. A paper by Martin Paulus, a Professor of Psychiatry at the University of California, San Diego, that I read shortly after it appeared in October, 2007, further reinforced the importance of homeostatic forces in psychological dysfunction. During a period of a few weeks after reading this paper, it became clear to me that the addictive drive and the homeostatic drive could be seen as opposing forces, and that this basic dynamic provided a unifying framework that could be used to understand all psychological health and dysfunction.

Another key development during this period was realizing that negative emotional states, such as the feeling of being "less than," create unconscious survival-mode states because they signal true survival risks in a hunter-gatherer context. All other distressing emotional states then also began to make sense when seen in this light. Viewing craving for food and sex as survival-mode states also made sense of findings that such states activate all the components of the so-called "stress" response and made it more clear how addictive payoffs could be distinguished from healthy payoffs. This then led to many of the ideas described in Chapters 1-6 and in the latter part of Chapter 7. During the next few months, I realized how the biological concept of homeostasis could be integrated with the classical, "spiritual" notion of the True Self. These ideas are woven throughout the book, but are described most explicitly in Chapters 14 and 15.

I want to express my gratitude to Richard Dobson, who shared with me his deep understanding of human psychology and spirituality. He and Ally Hamilton also introduced me to some of the "enlightenment" figures and literature that significantly shifted my own orientation. Two years or so before I began the work described in this book, both Ally and Richard also independently suggested, during conversations with me, that many people seem to be deriving some sort of reward from their own distress and pain.

David Anderson, my principal adviser while I was a graduate student at Caltech, and John Allman, who was on my thesis committee at Caltech and with whom I had frequent conversations, taught me an enormous amount about how to theorize, think, and do research. I was deeply influenced, in particular, by John's evolutionary approach to behavior. I also vividly recall the day he told me that hunter-gatherers were extraordinarily healthy physically. I feel very fortunate to have been trained by such world-class talents. Kent Berridge's work has also influenced me greatly, and I'm extremely grateful for his gracious support of my own work.

Jiro Tanaka made several helpful comments on a portion of this manuscript, and also made a number of helpful suggestions about the book layout and cover design. Jiro also gave me some invaluable general advice about writing that I'll never forget. My brother Geoff has taught me a great deal and generously shared with me his deep knowledge about writing when I first started doing journalism.

Sharon Fagen has always supported me in whatever I've chosen to do. It would be impossible for me to adequately express, in words, my gratitude for her love, generosity, kindness, and friendship. Helen Shardray has been a pleasure to work with and I am very grateful to her for all of her help. Thanks also to Noel Rowe for kindly allowing us to use the photograph of the lemur that's on the cover. I would also like to particularly thank Terry Bulych, Marilina Camacho, Allyson Chase, Raffaella D'Auria, Linda Davidson, Manijeh Ghaffari, Ali Grace, Kristen Hudson, Julie Jaskol, Denise Maratos, Alexis Markowitz, Vickie Rubin, Ellen Vash, Volee Young, Foojan Zeine, and my family for all of their help and support during this long process.

John Montgomery
Santa Monica, CA
March, 2010

NOTES

Many additional references that discuss the neuroscience, psychology, and anthropology research referred to in this book can be found in the text, notes, and bibliography of *The Answer Model Theory*.

Introduction

p. 5 **Researchers have found that stress hormones such as cortisol have effects in the brain that are almost identical to the effects of addictive drugs like cocaine.** Koob, G. F. 2008. A role for brain stress systems in addiction. *Neuron 59*, 11-34; Piazza, P. V., & Le Maol, M. 1997. Glucocorticoids as a biological substrate of reward: physiological and pathophysiological implications. *Brain Research Reviews 25*, 359-372; Montgomery, J. & Ritchey, T. 2008. *The Answer Model Theory*. Santa Monica, CA: TAM Books.

p. 6-7 **The ultimate goal of all psychotherapy, and of all emotional and psychological healing, as the psychologist Carl Jung said, is the dissolution of the false self and the discovery of the True Self.** Jung, C. G. 1966. *The spirit in man, art, and literature*. Princeton, NJ: Princeton University Press

p. 8 **Our view of addiction is very similar to what Buddhists call "attachment."** Note that the Buddhist use of the word "attachment" – perhaps an unfortunate and misleading English translation that confuses a Buddhist notion – is quite different from the common use of the word suggesting love and emotional connection. The use of the word in Buddhism is also quite different from its use by "attachment" theorists in modern psychology. See also Suzuki, D. T. 1960. *Manual of Zen Buddhism*. New York: Grove Press; Rahula, W. 1959. *What the Buddha taught*. New York: Grove Press

p. 8 **Carl Jung, for example, believed that Buddhism is essentially inaccessible to Westerners** e.g. see Jung's foreword in: Suzuki, D. T. 1964. *An introduction to Zen Buddhism*. New York: Grove Weidenfeld

Chapter 1

p. 12 **Addictive drugs like cocaine and methamphetamine actually create many of their effects in the brain by triggering a massive stress response** Koob, G. F. 2008. A role for brain stress systems in addiction. *Neuron 59*, 11-34; Montgomery, J. & Ritchey, T. 2008. *The Answer Model Theory*. Santa Monica, CA: TAM Books

p. 12 **Sexual desire, for example, activates all the components of the so-called "stress" response** Nesse, R. M., & Young, E. A. 2000. Evolutionary origins and functions of the stress response. *Encyclopedia of Stress 2*, 79-84

p. 13 **But the apparent reason that endorphins evolved to be part of the stress response is that endorphins are potent analgesics** Kandel, E. R., Schwartz, J. H., & Jessell, T. M. (Eds.) 1991. *Principles of neural science, Third Edition*. New York: Elsevier pp. 397-398

p. 16   Studies have shown, for example, that when people have drinks that are secretly laced with methamphetamine, they may strongly prefer this drink to another similar drink without the methamphetamine Hart, C. L., Ward, A. S., Haney, M., Foltin, R. W., & Fischman, M. W. 2001. Methamphetamine self-administration by humans. *Psychopharmacology 157*, 75-81

pp. 14-19 **Activation of reward system by pleasurable and painful stimuli** Montgomery, J. & Ritchey, T. 2008. *The Answer Model Theory*. Santa Monica, CA: TAM Books. pp. 9-12

p. 17   **When war veterans with post-traumatic stress disorder are shown films with reenactments of war scenes that trigger their own war traumas, many of them have powerful emotional responses** Pitman, R. K., van der Kolk, B. A., Orr, S. P., & Greenberg, M. S. 1990. Naloxone-reversible analgesic response to combat-related stimuli in posttraumatic stress disorder: A pilot study. *Arch Gen Psychiatry 47(6)*, 541-544

Chapter 2

pp. 22-23 **Release of dopamine and endorphin by hunger for food and sexual desire** Montgomery, J. & Ritchey, T. 2008. *The Answer Model Theory*. Santa Monica, CA: TAM Books. pp. 23-24

pp. 26-28 **Anxiety and depression** Montgomery, J. & Ritchey, T. 2008. *The Answer Model Theory*. Santa Monica, CA: TAM Books. pp. 20-21

p. 30   **Dopamine receptor levels and stress** Montgomery, J. & Ritchey, T. 2008. *The Answer Model Theory*. Santa Monica, CA: TAM Books. p. 17

Chapter 3

pp. 33-44 **"Less than" and addiction** Montgomery, J. & Ritchey, T. 2008. *The Answer Model Theory*. Santa Monica, CA: TAM Books. pp. 29-30

pp. 37-40 **Hunter-gatherers and status** Montgomery, J. & Ritchey, T. 2008. *The Answer Model Theory*. Santa Monica, CA: TAM Books. pp. 31-34

p. 42   **But the same brain imaging study showed that a loss in status also activates reward areas** Zink, C. F., Tong, Y., Chen, Q., Bassett, D. S., Stein, J. L., & Meyer-Lindenberg, A. 2008. Know your place: Neural processing of social hierarchy in humans. *Neuron 58*, 273-283

Chapter 4

pp. 45-54 **Parenting and addiction** Montgomery, J. & Ritchey, T. 2008. *The Answer Model Theory*. Santa Monica, CA: TAM Books. pp. 26-28

p. 47   **Stress and psychological dysfunction** Montgomery, J. & Ritchey, T. 2008. *The Answer Model Theory*. Santa Monica, CA: TAM Books. p. 25

Chapter 5

p. 55   **People who have undergone severe trauma, such as repeated sexual abuse, can become extraordinarily disconnected from their bodily experience** van der Kolk, B. A. 2003. Posttraumatic stress disorder and the nature of trauma. In M. F. Solomon & D. J. Siegel (Eds.), *Healing Trauma: attachment, mind, body, and brain*. New York: W. W. Norton

p. 56   **Many studies have suggested that the brain, at least in large part, creates emotional states by interpreting changes in the state of the body** Damasio, A. R. 1994. *Descartes' error*. New York: Avon Books; Craig, A. D. 2002. How do you feel? Interoception: the sense of the physiological condition of the body. *Nature Reviews Neuroscience 3*, 655-666

p. 57   **Physical and sexual abuse of children is extremely rare in hunter-gatherers** Hewlett, B. S., & Lamb, M. E (Eds.), *Hunter-gatherer childhoods*. New Jersey: Transaction Publishers

p. 58   **Mbuti pygmies** Turnbull, C. M. 1965. *Wayward servants: The two worlds of the African Pygmies*. New York: Natural History Press p. 142

p. 60   "If things cannot go straight, they will have to go crooked." Jung, C. G. 1982. *Aspects of the feminine*. Princeton, NJ: Princeton University Press p. 63

Chapter 6

p. 65   **anything that affects the body will also affect the mind, since the brain contains elaborate maps that are constantly monitoring and responding to the state of the body** Craig, A. D. 2002. How do you feel? Interoception: the sense of the physiological condition of the body. *Nature Reviews Neuroscience 3*, 655-666

p. 66   **Social isolation in modern life is well known to be a major risk factor for various neuroses and psychopathologies** Montgomery, J. & Ritchey, T. 2008. *The Answer Model Theory*. Santa Monica, CA: TAM Books. pp. 50-54

p. 66   **All animals that experience a survival threat will have a number of character-istic responses in their bodies** Estes, R. D. 1991. *The behavior guide to African mammals*. Los Angeles: University of California Press

p. 67   **But when the stress system is activated chronically, it can lead to high blood pressure and various heart conditions like atherosclerosis** Sapolsky, R. M. 2004. *Why zebras don't get ulcers*. New York: Henry Holt

p. 67   **Studies have shown that hunter-gatherers almost never develop high blood pressure** Eaton, S. B., & Eaton, S. B. III. 1999. Hunter-gatherers and human health. In Lee, R. B., & Daly, R. (Eds.), *The Cambridge encyclopedia of hunters and gatherers*. Cambridge, UK: Cambridge University Press

p. 67   **Nearly all animals raise their shoulders and scrunch their neck downwards when threatened with attack** Estes, R. D. 1991. *The behavior guide to African mammals*. Los Angeles: University of California Press

p. 70   **When we go into survival mode, our breathing becomes agitated** Sapolsky, R. M. 2004. *Why zebras don't get ulcers*. New York: Henry Holt

p. 71   While foregoing digestion can help an animal or person to survive during a true emergency, chronic, addiction-driven stomach disturbances can have ruinous effects on the digestive tract Sapolsky, R. M. 2004. *Why zebras don't get ulcers*. New York: Henry Holt

p. 72   The immune system has a complicated response in survival emergencies Sapolsky, R. M. 2004. *Why zebras don't get ulcers*. New York: Henry Holt

p. 72   The immune system and cancer Raulet, D. H. & Guerra, N. 2009. Oncogenic stress sensed by the immune system: Role of natural killer cell receptors. *Nature Reviews Immunology 9*, 568-580

Chapter 7

p. 78   The psychiatrist Albert Moll, for example, used hypnosis to show how people can readily create justifications for even the most bizarre behavior Wegner, D. M. 2002. *The illusion of conscious will*. Cambridge, MA: The MIT Press p. 150

p. 81   Flow states: Csikszentmihalyi, M. 1990. *Flow*. New York: Harper Perennial

p. 83   All animals, including humans, revert to old ingrained patterns when survival is at risk Panksepp, J. 1998. Affective neuroscience. New York: Oxford University Press; Dias-Ferreira, E. et. al. 2009. Chronic stress causes frontostriatal reorganization and affects decision-making. *Science 325*, 621-625

p. 84   Multiple Personality Disorder Schreiber, F. R. 1973. Sybil. New York: Warner Books; Dorahy, M. J. 2001. Dissociative identity disorder and memory dysfunction: The current state of experimental research and its future directions. *Clinical Psychology Review 21(5)*, 771-795

p. 86   The general rule in the brain is "use it or lose it." Doidge, N. 2007. *The brain that changes itself*. New York: Penguin

Chapter 8

p. 88   As the observers either watch the electric shocks being delivered, or if they themselves administer the electric shocks, reward areas in their brains become strongly activated De Quervain, D. J. F., Fischbacher, U., Treyer, V., Schellhammer, M., Schnyder, U., Buck, A., & Fehr, E. 2004. The neural basis of altruistic punishment. *Science 305*, 1254-1258; Singer, T., Seymour, B., O'Doherty, J. P., Stephan, K. E., Dolan, R. J., & Frith, C. D. 2006. Empathic neural responses are modulated by the perceived fairness of others. *Nature 439*, 466-469; Montgomery, J. & Ritchey, T. 2008. *The Answer Model Theory*. Santa Monica, CA: TAM Books. p. 39

p. 90   Women who suffer through chronic abuse, for example, have almost always been seriously abused as children van der Kolk, B. A. 2005. Child abuse & victimization. *Psychiatric Annals 35(5)*, 374-378

p. 92   One useful system for analyzing dysfunctional relationship interactions views the interactions as "control dramas." Redfield, J. 1993. *The Celestine prophecy*. New York: Warner Books pp. 126-130

Chapter 9

p. 100   Chimpanzees who are put in a cage alone will often bite their own leg until the leg bleeds Brüne, M., Brüne-Cohrs, U., McGrew, W. C., Preuschoft, S. 2006. Psychopathology in great apes: Concepts, treatment options and possible homologies to human psychiatric disorders. *Neuroscience and Biobehavioral Reviews 30*, 1246-1259

p. 101   "To the question 'What use are you making of your talents?' he answers, 'This thing stops me; I cannot go ahead,' and points to his self-erected barricade." Adler, A. (Ansbacher, H. L. & Ansbacher, R. R. Eds). 1956. *The individual psychology of Alfred Adler*. New York: HarperPerennial p. 265

p. 104   The common notion, even among medical professionals, that drug addiction is an essentially incurable genetic "disease" Peele, S. 2004. *7 tools to beat addiction*. New York: Three Rivers Press

p. 105   There is no precedent in our genetic or hunter-gatherer heritage for our being substance abusers or alcoholics Sullivan, R. J., & Hagen, E. H. 2002. Psychotropic substance-seeking: evolutionary pathology or adaptation? *Addiction 97*, 389-400

Chapter 10

p. 108   Studies have shown, for example, that giving money to charitable organizations strongly activates reward centers Harbaugh, W. T., Mayr, U., & Burghart, D. R. 2007. Neural responses to taxation and voluntary giving reveal motives for charitable donations. *Science 316*, 1622-1625

p. 111   Persistent pain, in turn, will almost always give rise to at least some anger Panksepp, J. 1998. *Affective neuroscience*. New York: Oxford University Press; Grandin, T. 2005. *Animals in translation*. New York: Harcourt p. 146;

p. 114   Some studies have suggested, for example, that at least one reason young mothers can develop Obsessive Compulsive Disorder, or even post-partum depression, is that they can't shake the obsessive thought of wanting to physically harm their babies Brandes, M., Soares, C. N., & Cohen L. S. 2004. Postpartum onset obsessive-compulsive disorder: Diagnosis and management. *Arch Womens Ment Health 7*, 99-110;

Chapter 11

p. 117   Millions of people have similar stories of events – we call them "life interventions" Peele, S. 2004. *7 tools to beat addiction*. New York: Three Rivers Press

Chapter 13

p. 129   **All humor and verbal banter are forms of play. Sports, art, literature, and music also arise, at least in large part, from this same ancient biological drive to play** Huizinga, J. 1950. *Homo ludens: A study of the play element in culture.* Boston: The Beacon Press; Burghardt, G. M. 2005. *The genesis of animal play.* Cambridge, MA: The MIT Press

p. 129   **if rats are exposed even briefly to the scent of a fox, their natural predator, the rats may not play for days** Panksepp, J. 1998. *Affective neuroscience.* New York: Oxford University Press

p. 130   **Many anthropologists have reported that games and play in hunter-gatherer cultures are largely non-competitive** Montgomery, J. & Ritchey, T. 2008. *The Answer Model Theory.* Santa Monica, CA: TAM Books. *pp. 47-49*

p. 134   **Dopamine, for example, is an important neurochemical not only for play and addiction, but also for dreaming** Montgomery, J. & Ritchey, T. 2008. *The Answer Model Theory.* Santa Monica, CA: TAM Books. *pp. 43-46*

p. 136   **Dream researchers like Kelly Bulkeley** Bulkeley, K. 2000. *Transforming dreams.* New York: John Wiley and Sons

p. 136   **"I experienced the incredible anguish of knowing my life was soon to end..."** Bulkeley, K. 2000. *Transforming dreams.* New York: John Wiley and Sons pp. 67-68

Chapter 14

p. 139   **All other animals, to varying degrees, seem to be far more tied to the present** Suddendorf, T., & Busby, J. 2003. Mental time travel in animals? *Trends in Cognitive Sciences 7(9),* 391-396

p. 139   **A key concept in Buddhism, as well as in many other major spiritual traditions, is the importance of living in the present moment** Rahula, W. 1959. *What the Buddha taught.* New York: Grove Press

p. 139   **While there has been a great deal of attention paid to living in the "present moment," or in the "Now,"** Tolle, E. 1999. *The power of now.* Novato, California: New World Library. While Tolle is clearly describing states that, in our terms, are "homeostatic" states, we are suggesting that focusing on "homeostasis," rather than the "Now," may be less prone to misinterpretation.

p. 143   **Studies have shown that when people are visualizing images in their minds called up from the past... they literally don't see what's in front of them as well as they normally would.** Ganis, G., Thompson, W. L., and Kosslyn, S. M. (2004). Brain areas underlying visual mental imagery and visual perception: an fMRI study. *Cognitive Brain Research, 20,* 226-24

Chapter 15

p. 144   **In the spiritual and enlightenment literature, particularly in Buddhism, there is much discussion about being fully "awake."** Tolle, E. 2005. *A new earth.* New York:

165

Dutton; Cohen, A. 2000. *Embracing heaven & earth.* Lenox, Massachusetts: Moksha Press; Rahula, W. 1959. *What the Buddha taught.* New York: Grove Press

p. 147   There's a long and somewhat complicated tradition in Christianity called Gnosticism that is also specifically concerned with the True Self Pagels, E. 1979. *The Gnostic gospels.* New York: Vintage; King, K. L. 2003. *What is Gnosticism?* Cambridge, Massachusetts: Harvard University Press; Jonas, H. 2001. *The Gnostic religion.* Boston: Beacon Press

p. 147   Carl Jung, who embraced the main tenets of Gnosticism, said that the True Self is the "God-image" within the human psyche Jung, C. G. 1958. *Psyche and Symbol.* Princeton, NJ: Princeton University Press

p. 148   Jung believed that while Christ was a true prophet, a deeply enlightened spiritual teacher of genius, Christ also became a symbol of the higher self Jung, C. G. 1958. *Psyche and Symbol.* Princeton, NJ: Princeton University Press

p. 148   The Buddha, for example, said that if he was a "God," then so too was every other human being Rahula, W. 1959. *What the Buddha taught.* New York: Grove Press

p. 148   Many scholars, such as Elaine Pagels... have argued that the core teachings of Jesus were very similar to the teachings of the Buddha Pagels, E. 1979. *The Gnostic gospels.* New York: Vintage

p. 148   But the disciples did not understand what Jesus meant, Jung said, and they took Jesus himself to be God Jung, C. G. 1997. *Visions Volume 1: Notes of the seminar given in 1930-1934.* Princeton, NJ: Princeton University Press p. 586

p. 148   "The Kingdom of God is within you," Luke 17:21

p. 148   "I am the way, the truth, and the life: no man cometh unto the Father, but by me" John 14:6

p. 148   But Carl Jung suggested that this statement actually refers to the True Self Jung, C. G. 1958. *Psyche and Symbol.* Princeton, NJ: Princeton University Press

NOTES

NOTES

ABOUT THE AUTHORS:

John Montgomery received his Ph.D. in neuroscience from Caltech in Pasadena, California and his B.A. in molecular genetics from Trinity College in Dublin, Ireland. The primary author of *The Answer Model Theory*, he has also written about science for the Washington Post and The Economist, largely about the interface between psychology and neuroscience. He is also a counselor who uses The Answer Model, which he co-developed with Todd Ritchey. He lives in Santa Monica, CA.

Todd Ritchey is an addiction specialist with over a decade of experience as an interventionist, counselor, and mentor. He has treated families and couples dealing with substance abuse, relationship issues, and a variety of other painful conditions and circumstances. The Answer Model method has proven to be extraordinarily effective for his clients. Todd lives in Vancouver, British Columbia, with his wife of twenty-four years and their three children.

CPSIA information can be obtained at www.ICGtesting.com
Printed in the USA
BVOW06s1726300716

457046BV00010B/89/P